Health

A Multimedia Source Guide

Health

A Multimedia Source Guide

by

Joan Ash

and

Michael Stevenson

R. R. Bowker Company
A Xerox Publishing Company
New York & London, 1976

Published by R. R. Bowker Company (a Xerox Publishing Company)
1180 Avenue of the Americas, New York, N.Y. 10036
Copyright © 1976 by Xerox Corporation
Printed and bound in the United States of America

Library of Congress Cataloging in Publication Data

Ash, Joan.
  Health: a multimedia source guide.
  Includes indexes.
    1. Hygiene—Audio-visual aids—Catalogs. 2. Health
education—Audio-visual aids—Catalogs. I. Stevenson,
Michael. II. Title.
RA440.55.Z9A83   613'.07   76-28297
ISBN 0-8352-0905-9

TO BRITT AND PAUL

Contents

Preface .... *ix*

Introduction .... *xi*

A. Associations, Societies, and Foundations *53*
B. Audiovisual Producers and Distributors *1*
C. Book Dealers *101*
D. City, State, and Federal Agencies *105*
E. Libraries and Information Services *115*
F. Pharmaceutical and Other Companies *131*
G. Publishers *139*
H. Research Institutes *161*

Source Index *165*
Index to Free or Inexpensive Material *175*
Subject Index *177*

Preface

Librarians are constantly faced with the patron eager to know more about a particular health problem or about the health status of a group or population. These questions are of a sensitive nature when self-diagnosis, treatment, interpretation, or distrust of the physician are involved. What materials should be on hand or requested, or to whom should such questions be referred?

As health professionals become more concerned with their patient-education function, they find an increasing need for a list of information sources catering to clients on all levels of education and experience. The intelligent layman himself often needs a handy book which will tell him where to go for information on the tuberculin test he was given at work, for a source of tactfully written sex information for his children, for a list of planned parenthood clinics, or for some free material for his daughter's term paper on the health hazards of mercury in the environment. The most helpful reference book to aid the librarian, health professional, and layman alike would provide, in one place, current, accurate, and succinct information on where to find these answers.

This volume is intended to serve the needs of all three groups (librarians, health professionals, and laymen). Because publications change and become dated, and because information takes many forms other than the printed word, this book is more than a list of published sources. It is an annotated guide to organizations which deal with health-related matters—publishers, audiovisual dealers and distributors, libraries, government agencies, societies (both professional and voluntary), pharmaceutical companies, book dealers, and research institutes.

The authors would like to thank all of the professional and personal friends who have aided in the compilation of this book. The generosity of those people who returned questionnaires is much appreciated. Madeliene Miele and Pat Schuman of the Bowker Company deserve special thanks, as does Pam Johnson who did the subject index. The staff at the Lyman Maynard Stowe Library of the University of Connecticut Health Center was extremely helpful in letting us use audiovisual and publishers' catalogs. Joan would like to express her loving appreciation for the encouragement, help, and tolerance of her husband Paul. Mike is particularly grateful for past help and interest from Jan Mathews, Bob Edwards, and Peter Martin.

Joan Ash
Michael Stevenson

Introduction

To compile *Health: A Multimedia Source Guide*, the authors sent questionnaires to over 3,000 agencies in the United States. This mailing list was generated by careful scanning of numerous printed directories such as *Encyclopedia of Associations, Health Sciences Libraries in the United States*. Among the questions asked were: Whom do you serve? Do you publish anything? What kinds of verbal information do you provide? Most significant was the request that the organization send along samples or descriptive material when returning the questionnaire.

About 500 questionnaires were returned, most with packets of additional material. If a second mailing did not generate a response from a particularly valuable source, other means of tracking down the information were sought. In this respect, the collections of publishers' and audiovisual producers' catalogs at the University of Connecticut Health Center Library were invaluable; sources traced by this means are designated by an asterisk. A total of approximately 700 groups or organizations are listed.

The authors have attempted to point out important facts about each information source without including details which the user of the volume can best obtain from the source itself. For example, in the Publishers section, emphasis is placed on general subject areas rather than on individual publications. The user who is interested in a general subject can request a catalog from the particular publisher.

Scope and Arrangement

Except for particularly important sources, like the Film Board of Canada or foreign publishers with large American distributing companies, only sources in the United States are included. Questionnaires were sent to national organizations with over five hundred members, again with a few exceptions. "Health," in this volume, is broadly interpreted to include not only medicine, dentistry, nursing, and public health, but also areas like engineering, physics, and other basic sciences which relate to health.

This volume is divided into eight sections according to type of source, each source having its own entry number. Cross references have been liberally included in the text, since many sources produce several types of information (for example, an association often publishes books and distributes audiovisuals or verbal information). Three indexes are provided. The first lists all seven hundred sources alphabetically, again with cross references. The second is an index to sources which provide free or inexpensive pamphlet material to the layman, and can serve as a resource guide for patient-education materials or pamphlet files. The third index lists sources by subject.

A

Associations, Societies, and Foundations

A1. ACADEMY OF PSYCHOSOMATIC MEDICINE, Box 1053, Mountainside, N.J. 07092. J. Campbell Howard, M.D., Exec. Dir.

PURPOSE. A medical society, devoted to promoting care for the psyche as well as the physical body. *Specialization:* psychosomatic medicine.
PUBLICATIONS. *Psychosomatics* (quarterly). Payment not required with order.

A2. ACTION ON SMOKING AND HEALTH (ASH), Box 19556, 2000 H St. N.W., Washington, D.C. 20006. *Tel:* (202) 659-4310. John F. Bauzhaf III, Exec. Dir.

PURPOSE. "To take legal action with regard to problem of smoking and protect rights of nonsmokers." *Specialization:* smoking and health problems.
PRODUCTS. Buttons, bumper stickers, signs, labels. Payment required with order.

A3. AEROSPACE MEDICAL ASSOCIATION, Washington National Airport, Washington, D.C. 20001. *Tel:* (202) 638-2190. Merrill H. Goodwin, M.D., Exec. Vice-Pres.

PURPOSE. Concerned with continuing medical education. *Specialization:* aerospace medicine.
MEMBERSHIP. *Requirements:* Limited to professionals working in or interested in aviation, space, and environmental medicine. *Dues:* $50/yr.
PUBLICATIONS. *Aviation, Space and Environmental Medicine.* Payment required with order.

A4. ALCOHOL AND DRUG PROBLEMS ASSOCIATION OF NORTH AMERICA, 1101 15 St. N.W., Suite 204, Washington, D.C. 20005. *Tel:* (202) 452-0990. Augustus H. Hewlett, Exec. Dir.

1

PURPOSE. A professional and service organization, representing a broad constituency working in alcoholism treatment and drug abuse treatment. Lobbies federal agencies, Congress, and other organizations. *Specialization:* alcoholism and drug abuse.
MEMBERSHIP. *Dues:* agency $200; program $300; individual $20. *Benefits:* newsletter, employment listings, malpractice insurance.
PUBLICATIONS. *Alcoholism Facilities Directory*; selected papers from association's annual meeting and North American Congress. Payment not required with order.

A5. ALEXANDER GRAHAM BELL ASSOCIATION, 3417 Volta Place N.W., Washington, D.C. 20007. *Tel:* (202) 337-5220. George W. Fellendorf, Exec. Dir.

PURPOSE. To promote teaching of speech, lip-reading, and use of residual hearing for the hearing impaired. Disseminates information on deafness. *Specialization:* deafness and hearing impairment.
MEMBERSHIP. *Dues:* $15.
SPECIAL INFORMATION SERVICES. Information on deafness for parents, professionals, and other interested persons. *Special collections:* 20,000 volumes on deafness; extensive collection of periodicals, pamphlets, and clipping files. *Languages:* English and Spanish.
PUBLICATIONS. *Volta Review* (journal), *World Traveler* (children's magazine). Books and reprints on hearing impairment, aphasia, audiology, communication skills, education, multiple handicaps, and guides for parents. Payment required with order.

A6. ALLERGY FOUNDATION OF AMERICA, 801 Second Avenue, New York, N.Y. 10017. *Tel:* (212) 684-7875. John R. Rague, Exec. Dir.

PURPOSE. To unite the public, medical profession, researchers, and public health workers in seeking to increase knowledge of causes and treatment for asthma and allergic diseases. *Specialization:* allergy.
SPECIAL INFORMATION SERVICES. Lists of allergists and clinics in all 50 states.
PUBLICATIONS. Pamphlets on the foundation and on allergies (12 pamphlets on hay fever, insect stings, and other allergies are available). Payment required with order.

A7. ALTON OCHSNER MEDICAL FOUNDATION, Department of Photography, 1514 Jefferson Hwy., New Orleans, La. 70121.* *Tel:* (504) 834-7070.

PURPOSE. A health foundation offering films to professionals. *Specialization:* medical films.
PUBLICATIONS. Films on surgical procedures and internal medicine (produced by Ochsner or by Davis & Geck).

A8. AMERICAN ACADEMY OF ALLERGY, 225 E. Michigan St., Milwaukee, Wis. 53202. *Tel:* (414) 272-6071. James O. Kelley, Exec. Dir.

PURPOSE. Concerned with postgraduate medical education.
MEMBERSHIP. *Requirements:* M.D., Ph.D. or foreign equivalent, and interest in allergy and clinical immunology.
PUBLICATIONS. *Journal of Allergy and Clinical Immunology* (monthly). Free to members; others may subscribe.

A9. AMERICAN ACADEMY OF CHILD PSYCHIATRY, 1800 R St. N.W., Suite 904, Washington, D.C. 20009. *Tel:* (202) 462-3754. Virginia Bausch, Exec. Sec.

PURPOSE. A central office for the representation of child psychiatrists. Publishes information on legislation, as well as scientific papers. *Specialization:* child psychiatry.
PUBLICATIONS. *Journal of the American Academy of Child Psychiatry* (quarterly); two yearly newsletters containing interoffice and committee information. Payment required with order.
INQUIRY ADDRESS. Yale University Press, 92-A Yale Station, New Haven, Conn. 06520. *Tel:* (203) 432-4973.

A10. AMERICAN ACADEMY OF DENTAL ELECTROSURGERY, INC., 57 W. 57 St., New York, N.Y. 10019. *Tel:* (212) 755-6630. Maurice J. Oringer, Exec. Sec.

PURPOSE. To promote the proper use of electrosurgery in dentistry through scientific programs, research, and publications. *Specialization:* uses of electrosurgery in dental disciplines.
MEMBERSHIP. *Requirements:* member in good standing of American Dental Association or foreign counterpart; five years clinical practice, instruction in dental electrosurgery. *Dues:* $35/yr.
SPECIAL INFORMATION SERVICES. Replies to inquiries by members in matters of academy's interests.
PUBLICATIONS. Monthly mimeographed newsletter.

A11. AMERICAN ACADEMY OF FORENSIC SCIENCES, 11400 Rockville Pike, Suite 515, Rockville, Md. 20852. *Tel:* (301) 881-0537. Margaret M. Hibbard, Exec. Dir.

PURPOSE. To promote education for and research in forensic science so that the criminal justice system will benefit from knowledge of law, medicine, and science.
MEMBERSHIP. *Requirements:* Professionals in the forensic sciences.
PUBLICATIONS. *Journal of Forensic Sciences* (quarterly); newsletter and roster.

A12. AMERICAN ACADEMY OF HEALTH ADMINISTRATION, National Office, East Texas State University, Texarkana, Tex. 75501. *Tel:* (214) 794-2569. Don C. Dodson, Exec. Dir.

PURPOSE. To improve management procedures and administrative practice of those involved in health services.
MEMBERSHIP. Open to anyone involved in performance, education, research, or generally concerned with management areas within health field. *Dues:* $10/yr.
PUBLICATIONS. Newsletter (annual), annual meeting proceedings, membership directory, pamphlets.

A13. AMERICAN ACADEMY OF OPHTHALMOLOGY AND OTOLARYNGOLOGY-CONTINUING EDUCATION WITH TELEVISION, c/o Visual Information Systems, 15 Columbus Circle, New York, N.Y. 10023. *Tel:* (212) 541-8080. Don Monaco, Coor.

PURPOSE. To produce and distribute videotape packages, providing comprehensive review for practicing ophthalmologists and otolaryngologists, emphasizing self-directed learning. (Services restricted to practicing physicians.) *Specialization:* opthalmology and otoloryngology.

PUBLICATIONS. Free catalogs describe 20 available programs in otolaryngology and 8 in ophthalmology. Each program has a 50-minute videocassette (available in all standard formats) oriented toward surgical and examination techniques. Otolaryngology series includes written supplementary material. Payment required with order (reduced rates for members).

INQUIRY ADDRESS. Mark Wein, AAOO-CETV, 15 Columbus Circle, New York, N.Y. 10023. *Tel:* (212) 541-8080.

A14. AMERICAN ACADEMY OF OPTOMETRY, 115 W. Broadway, Box 566, Owatonna, Minn. 55060. *Tel:* 451-0009. John N. Schoen, Sec.-Treas.

PURPOSE. To further development of optometrical sciences. *Specialization:* optometry-optometrics.

MEMBERSHIP. *Requirements:* graduate optometrist or visual scientist and meet admissions requirements. *Dues:* $20–$40.

PUBLICATIONS. *American Journal of Optometry and Physiological Optics* (monthly). Payment not required with order.

A15. AMERICAN ACADEMY OF ORAL PATHOLOGY, Ohio State University College of Dentistry, Columbus, Ohio 43210. *Tel:* (614) 422-1421. Dr. George F. Blozis, Sec.-Treas.

PURPOSE. A professional society organized to exchange scientific information.

MEMBERSHIP. *Requirements:* interest in oral pathology. *Dues:* $37. *Benefits:* members receive publications and may attend annual meeting.

PRODUCTS. Microscopic slides and color transparencies. Some selections may only be ordered by members. Payment required with order.

A16. AMERICAN ACADEMY OF ORTHOPAEDIC SURGEONS, 430 N. Michigan Ave., Chicago, Ill. 60611. *Tel:* (312) 822-0970. Charles V. Heck, M.D., Exec. Dir.

PURPOSE. To provide continuing education for orthopedic surgeons and allied professionals. *Specialization:* orthopedic surgery and emergency care.

MEMBERSHIP. *Requirements:* only board-certified orthopedic surgeons.

PUBLICATIONS. One-hundred-page visual aids index listing sound-slide and film selections with suggested audience. Aimed at children, adults, general audiences, residents, and orthopedists. Includes lively and readable discussion of how to produce an instructive film. Majority of books and films cover surgery and diagnosis; care and transportation of sick and injured also treated. Payment required with order.

A17. AMERICAN ACADEMY OF OSTEOPATHY, 2630 Airport Rd., Colorado Springs, Colo. 80910. *Tel:* (303) 632-7164. Louise W. Astell, Dir.

PURPOSE. To provide continuing medical education to osteopathic physicians with emphasis on palpatory diagnosis and manipulative treatment of neuromusculoskeletal system. (Services restricted to members of the academy, the osteopathic profession, medical doctors, dentists, and optometrists.) *Specialization:* neuro-musculoskeletal system.

MEMBERSHIP. *Requirements:* must be member of American Osteopathic Association. *Dues:* $35. *Benefits:* Members receive yearbook, newsletter, and other publications.

PUBLICATIONS. Yearbook, quarterly newsletter, reprints, and original articles. Payment preferred with order.

A18. AMERICAN ACADEMY OF PEDIATRICS, 1801 Hinman Ave., Evanston, Ill. 60204. *Tel:* (312) 869-4255. Robert Frazier, M.D., Exec. Dir.

PURPOSE. "The attainment by all children of the Americas of their full potential for physical, emotional, and social health." *Specialization:* pediatrics.

MEMBERSHIP. *Requirements:* members must be certified by American Board of Pediatrics. *Dues:* $100/yr. *Benefits:* members receive all academy publications free, reduced meeting rates, insurance packages.

PUBLICATIONS. Manuals on infectious diseases, school health, retardation, and other topics, $3/single copy. Pamphlets and reprints on large and varied selection of topics: poisoning, accidents, athletics, nutrition, disabilities, youth. (Bulk rates available) *Pediatrics* (monthly), $17/yr. for nonmembers. *News and Comments* (monthly), free. Reprints of committee statements from these periodicals can be ordered separately. Payment required with order.

A19. AMERICAN ASSOCIATION FOR CANCER RESEARCH, 7701 Burholme Ave., Fox Chase, Philadelphia, Pa. 19111. *Tel:* (215) FI 2-1000, Ext. 420. Hugh J. Creech, Sec.-Treas.

PURPOSE. To arrange annual meeting for presentation of research results and publication of monthly journal through subsidiary, Cancer Research, Inc. *Specialization:* cancer research.

MEMBERSHIP. *Requirements:* nomination by two active members; must have published two papers.

PUBLICATIONS. *Cancer Research* (monthly), $75/yr. for nonmembers. Payment required with order.

A20. AMERICAN ASSOCIATION FOR MATERNAL AND CHILD HEALTH, INC., Box 965, Los Altos, Calif. 94022. *Tel:* (415) 964-4575. Harold J. Fishbein, Exec. Dir.

PURPOSE. To promote maternal and child health by bringing together health professionals and the people they serve. *Specialization:* maternal and child health.

MEMBERSHIP. Professionals, administrators, and consumers in medical-dental fields.

PUBLICATIONS. Booklets and reprints for professionals and lay people on child care, pregnancy, nutrition, nursing babies, safety, and diseases. Ten sound filmstrips on similar subjects. Payment not required with institutional order.

A21. THE AMERICAN ASSOCIATION FOR THE ABOLITION OF INVOL-UNTARY HOSPITALIZATION, INC., Post Office, University of Santa Clara, Santa Clara, Calif. 95053. George F. Alexander, Chmn.

PURPOSE. To abolish involuntary hospitalization.
MEMBERSHIP. *Dues:* $10/yr.
SPECIAL INFORMATION SERVICES. Aid to those needing legal assistance.
PUBLICATIONS. Periodicals. Payment required with order.

A22. AMERICAN ASSOCIATION FOR THE ADVANCEMENT OF SCIENCE, 1515 Massachusetts Ave. N.W., Washington, D.C. 20005.*

PURPOSE. To organize professionals and others interested in promoting scientific endeavors in all fields, from medicine to space flight. *Specialization:* information in all areas of science.
MEMBERSHIP. *Dues:* $25/yr.
PUBLICATIONS. *Science* (weekly); *Science Books and Films* (quarterly) (for teachers), reviews materials recently released, for all educational levels. Audiotape programs; symposia recorded in print and on tape. Payment not required with order.

A23. AMERICAN ASSOCIATION FOR WORLD HEALTH, INC. (U.S. Committee for the World Health Organization), 777 United Nations Plaza, No. 9A, New York, N.Y. 10017. *Tel:* (212) 986-8451. Philip E. Nelbach, Exec. Vice-Pres.

PURPOSE. To inform Americans about world health problems, and to interest them in and assist the work of WHO and other agencies toward solving these problems.
MEMBERSHIP. *Dues:* individual $15/yr.; libraries $25/yr.; organizations $250/yr.
SPECIAL INFORMATION SERVICES. Inquiries by nonmembers relative to literature or job opportunities will be answered if self-addressed, stamped envelope is enclosed.
PUBLICATIONS. WHO magazine *World Health*; PAHO magazine *Gazette*; U.S. Agency for International Development publications (available to members only).

A24. AMERICAN ASSOCIATION OF BIOANALYSTS, 411 N. Seventh St., Suite 805, St. Louis, Mo. 63101. *Tel:* (314) 241-1445. David Birenbaum, Admin.

PURPOSE. To foster and expand scientific, economic, and public health interests of bioanalytical laboratory directors and supervisors; to safeguard their economic interests; and to establish proper professional ethics for those engaged in the profession. (Services restricted to persons interested in clinical laboratory science.) *Specialization:* clinical laboratory science.
MEMBERSHIP. *Requirements:* owners, directors, and supervisors of independent bioanalytical laboratories. *Dues:* $60–$200/yr.
SPECIAL INFORMATION SERVICES. *Special collections:* slide library on health.
PUBLICATIONS. Pamphlets and periodicals. Bimonthly bulletin of developments in the field, "Test of the Month" series to study developments in laboratory disciplines. Proficiency Testing Service for internal quality control. Payment required with order.

A25. AMERICAN ASSOCIATION OF BLOOD BANKS, 1828 L St. N.W., Washington, D.C. 20036. *Tel:* (202) 872-8333. Robert Thomas, Exec. Dir.

PURPOSE. *Specialization:* blood banks.
MEMBERSHIP. *Requirements:* must meet standards of association and pay dues.
PUBLICATIONS. Books, pamphlets, films, slides, audio- and videotapes, and news

briefs; proceedings of seminars and meetings on transfusion, immunology, genetics, compatibility testing, antigens, hepatitis, freezing, and administration. Payment required with order.

A26. AMERICAN ASSOCIATION OF COLLEGES OF PHARMACY, 8121 Georgia Ave., Silver Spring, Md. 20910.*

PURPOSE. An association of institutions that trains professional pharmacists, promoting high standards of training and publishing information on careers in the field. *Specialization:* pharmacy.
PUBLICATIONS. *American Journal of Pharmaceutical Education* (five issues per year), $10/yr.; *AACP News* (monthly), $5/yr. to nonmembers, free to members. Rosters of teachers in colleges of pharmacy issued every other year. Sound/filmstrip program on careers for qualified pharmacists, $20. Other pamphlets on similar topics, as well as list of professional requirements, admissions requirements of schools, and bibliography of theses and dissertations in pharmacy administration (750 entries), $3. Payment not required with order.

A27. AMERICAN ASSOCIATION OF DENTAL SCHOOLS, 1625 Massachusetts Ave., Washington, D.C. 20036. *Tel:* (202) 667-9433. Dr. Harry W. Bruce, Jr., Exec. Dir.

PURPOSE. To improve dental education. *Specialization:* dental education.
MEMBERSHIP. *Requirements:* institutional—accredited dental schools and dental education programs, including auxiliary programs; individual—persons with demonstrable interest in dental education, dental students, and honorary members.
PUBLICATIONS. *Journal of Dental Education* (monthly); *Bulletin of Dental Education* (monthly newsletter); *Dental Student News* (bimonthly, October–May); *Proceedings* (annual report of annual session activities); *Directory of Dental Educators*, material on dental school admissions requirements, careers in dentistry, and salary survey. Pamphlet on membership. Payment required with noninstitutional order.

A28. AMERICAN ASSOCIATION OF DOCTORS' NURSES, 9600 Colesville Rd., Silver Spring, Md. 20901. *Tel:* (301) 585-1056. Bob Bickford, Exec. Dir.

PURPOSE. To promote education, training, welfare, and attitudes of the employee of the physician.
PRODUCTS. Antismoking stickers, $3/1,000.

A29. AMERICAN ASSOCIATION OF FOREIGN MEDICAL GRADUATES, 292 Madison Ave., New York, N.Y. 10017. *Tel:* (212) 949-5957. Hugh P. Curley, Exec. Sec.

PURPOSE. Primarily to "secure for the foreign medical graduate a general climate and atmosphere conducive to the achievement of his full potential" by promoting full assimilation, interracial and intercultural relations, better understanding of the foreign medical graduate, and financial aid.
MEMBERSHIP. *Requirements:* all graduates of foreign medical schools are eligible if they are licensed to practice medicine in the U.S. Unlicensed foreign medical graduates may also apply. *Dues:* $12/yr.; interns and residents $6/yr.

PUBLICATIONS. *Career Development for Foreign Medical Graduates in the United States,* a handbook by Dr. Yvan Silva, $4.75. A brochure entitled "Questions and Answers for Foreign Medical Graduates" and a bimonthly newsletter, *The Sentinel,* are available with membership. Payment required with order.
SPECIAL INFORMATION SERVICES. Information available on visa requirements, ECFMG and Flex exams.

A30. THE AMERICAN ASSOCIATION OF ORTHODONTISTS, 7477 Delmar Blvd., St. Louis, Mo. 63130. *Tel:* (314) 726-5616. James E. Brophy, Exec. Dir.

PURPOSE. To advance the science and art of orthodontics through encouraging and sponsoring research, and to strive for higher standards in orthodontics.
MEMBERSHIP. *Requirements:* must have training in and maintain practice in orthodontics.
SPECIAL INFORMATION SERVICES. Informational materials to members and lay educational groups, health clubs, others. *Special collections:* Charles R. Baker Memorial Library for members' use and audiovisual library that loans to academia, clubs, and members.
PUBLICATIONS. Colorful, explanatory morale-boosters for young and adult orthodontics patients. Manual on health-care programs in orthodontics; brochures on tooth brushing with braces; careers in field; bad habits that lead to malocclusions; posters. Also films, slides, and periodicals.

A31. AMERICAN ASSOCIATION OF SEX EDUCATORS AND COUNSEL-ORS, 5010 Wisconsin Ave. N.W., Suite 304, Washington, D.C. 20016. *Tel:* (202) 686-2523. Dr. Patricia Schiller, Chief Exec. Off.

PURPOSE. To establish sound basis for teaching of sex education and practice of sex therapy. *Specialization:* sex education and therapy.
MEMBERSHIP. *Requirements:* members must be involved in sex education and counseling or be students in those fields. *Dues:* $10–$20.
PUBLICATIONS. *Journal of Sex Education and Therapy* (semiannual); training manuals and books; booklets on adolescent sex, marriage counseling, sex and culture, sex and Jews, and family planning; newsletter. (Price lists available) Payment required with order.

A32. AMERICAN ASSOCIATION OF SUICIDOLOGY, Department of Psychiatry, Baylor Medical College, Houston, Tex. 77025. Dr. Richard McGee, Pres.

PURPOSE. A multidisciplinary organization of professionals and concerned lay people. Provides a forum for mutual discussion of suicidology. Organizes annual meetings devoted to research and suicide-prevention services. Develops standards and accreditation procedures for suicide-prevention centers.
PUBLICATIONS. *Suicide,* official journal; *Newslink,* newsletter; *Directory of Suicide Prevention Centers*; and specialized publications.
INQUIRY ADDRESS. Betsy S. Comstock, M.D., Sec., Department of Psychiatry, Baylor Medical College, Houston, Tex. 77025.

A33. AMERICAN BAR ASSOCIATION, Division of Communications, 1155 E. 60 St., Chicago, Ill. 60637.* *Tel:* (312) 493-0533. Harriet Wilson Ellis, Staff Dir., Audiovisual Department.

PURPOSE. A professional and regulatory organization of the legal profession in the United States. Producer of audiovisual programs on law for general public and members of the legal profession. *Specialization:* audiovisual programs on legal issues.
PUBLICATIONS. Eighty-page catalog (irregular), listing over 800 films and filmstrips in law, including distributors from which to rent and buy. Also includes series of six films coproduced by AMA and ABA on medicolegal issues. Large selection on drugs and the law and their physical effects, and selection on criminal psychopathology, as well as alcoholism. Payment depends on distributor of particular item.

A34. AMERICAN CANCER SOCIETY, 219 E. 42 St., New York, N.Y. 10017.* *Tel:* (212) 867-3700.

PURPOSE. A charitable organization supporting research and public information on cancer. *Specialization:* cancer.
PUBLICATIONS. Films for nurses and physicians on diagnosis and treatment, instructional aids for schoolteachers, public information via brochures and films. Publications on living with disease, cancer in children, and rehabilitation after treatment. Extensive list of publications and productions. Much of material is free.

A35. AMERICAN CHEMICAL SOCIETY, 1155 16 St. N.W., Washington, D.C. 20036. *Tel:* (202) 872-4600. Robert W. Cairns, Exec. Dir.

PURPOSE. To encourage advancement of chemistry in all its branches. *Specialization:* all fields of chemistry.
PUBLICATIONS. Journals of *Biochemistry, Environmental Science and Technology, Medicinal Chemistry,* and *Agricultural and Food Chemistry.* Thirty-four-page catalog of books, including symposia results, monographs, texts, indexes, reprints, and directories to chemical education. Short audiotape-and-slide courses. Payment not required with order.

A36. AMERICAN CHIROPRACTIC ASSOCIATION, 2200 Grand Ave., Des Moines, Iowa 50312. *Tel:* (515) 243-1121. Louis O. Gearhart, D.C., Exec. Dir.

PURPOSE. An association for professional, educational, and research services. *Specialization:* chiropractic.
MEMBERSHIP. *Requirements:* medical professionals licensed to practice chiropractic medicine.
SPECIAL INFORMATION SERVICES. Information on general health, safety, good posture, spinal disorders and care, and careers.
PUBLICATIONS. Pamphlets, *Chiropractic State of the Art,* and *Charter Provisions and Bylaws.* Also books, films, slides, records, and videotapes. *ACA Journal of Chiropractic* (monthly), $12.50/yr. Payment required with order.

A37. AMERICAN COLLEGE HEALTH ASSOCIATION, 2807 Central St., Evanston, Ill. 60201. *Tel:* (312) 491-9775. James W. Dilley, Exec. Dir.

PURPOSE. An organization of institutions of higher education and individuals promoting health for students and other members of college communities. *Specialization:* college and university health programs.

SPECIAL INFORMATION SERVICES. Uniform reporting program of costs and utilization of college and university health services.

PUBLICATIONS. Pamphlets, audiotapes, and periodicals. Payment required with order.

A38. AMERICAN COLLEGE OF CARDIOLOGY EXTENDED LEARNING, 9650 Rockville Pike, Bethesda, Md. 20014.*

PURPOSE. A professional organization offering materials on cardiology. *Specialization:* cardiovascular diseases.

PUBLICATIONS. Journal; audio- and videotapes available to physicians treating cardiovascular disease. Much offered on acupuncture.

A39. AMERICAN COLLEGE OF NURSE-MIDWIVES, 1000 Vermont Ave. N.W., No. 500, Washington, D.C. 20005. *Tel:* (202) 628-4642. Dorothea L. Russell, Exec. Sec.

PURPOSE. An association devoted to establishing standards, evaluating services, and promoting research in the field of nurse-midwifery. Promotes communication among practicing nurse-midwives, as well as between them and allied medical professionals. *Specialization:* nurse-midwifery.

MEMBERSHIP. *Requirements:* must be certified midwife. Active, associate, and student memberships.

PUBLICATIONS. *Journal of Nurse-Midwifery* (quarterly). Pamphlets and booklets on qualifications, programs, legislation, and data pertaining to education and practice of midwifery. Also delivery record book and set of 35mm slides that can be rented. Payment required with order.

A40. AMERICAN COLLEGE OF RADIOLOGY, 20 N. Wacker Dr., Chicago, Ill. 60606.* *Tel:* (312) 236-4963.

PURPOSE. A professional organization of radiologists. *Specialization:* radiology.

PUBLICATIONS. Twenty-two-page catalog covering fields of education, science, public relations, business, and government. For members, monthly newsletter and annual directory of members. For members and other professionals, results of symposia, self-evaluation programs, business practices, syllabi, indexes, manuals on Roentgen diagnosis, technologists' guides, and dangers of X-rays and other radiation. Booklets explaining radiological procedures to patients. Films for professionals showing diagnostic procedures and for patients showing radiologists at work. Slide sets, accompanied by syllabi and/or taped commentary, concentrating on mammography. Reprints on business procedures, X-ray technology, professional standards, and calibration of equipment. Payment required with order.

A41. AMERICAN COLLEGE OF SURGEONS, 55 E. Erie St., Chicago, Ill. 60611. *Tel:* (312) 664-4050. C. Rollins Hanlon, M.D., Dir.

PURPOSE. A professional organization of surgeons devoted to improving the quality of care for the surgical patient by elevating the standards of surgical education and practice. *Specialization:* surgery.

MEMBERSHIP. *Requirements:* must give concrete evidence of surgical education, surgical competence, and ethical fitness.

PUBLICATIONS. *Surgery, Gynecology and Obstetrics,* journal (monthly); *Surgical Forum* (annual). Limited-distribution periodicals are *Bulletin of the ACS* and *Yearbook.* Booklets, manuals, reprints on trauma and cancer, and OR Environment reports also published. Two patient-education reprints, one with Spanish translation. Catalogs of audiotapes and films on trauma. Single copies free; bulk rates on request.

A42. AMERICAN COLLEGE OF SURGEONS, Surgical Film Library, Davis & Geck Distributor, 1 Casper St., Danbury, Conn. 06810.

PURPOSE. A joint effort between the American College of Surgeons and the Davis & Geck Division of American Cyanamid Co. Distributes 16mm films on all aspects of surgery for the use of medical societies and their auxiliaries, medical schools, hospitals, and other groups of health sciences professionals. *Specialization:* surgery and nursing.

PUBLICATIONS. One-hundred-and-forty-page looseleaf catalog (complete with loose-leaf notebook) describes film offerings and will allow supplements to be added as they appear. Catalog is attractive guide to the 1,167 subjects offered, the largest selections being in cardiovascular systems, digestion, and operating room techniques. Each film is described as to course the surgery depicted takes, symptoms of subject, corrective action taken by surgeon/author, and postoperative results. Films are loaned to eligible groups, $7.50 for surgical films, $5 for nursing films. Payment not required with order.

INQUIRY ADDRESS. John M. Beal, M.D., F.A.C.S., Chmn., Committee on Medical Motion Pictures, American College of Surgeons, 55 E. Erie St., Chicago, Ill. 60611.

A43. AMERICAN CONGRESS OF REHABILITATION MEDICINE, 30 N. Michigan Ave., Chicago, Ill. 60602. *Tel:* (312) 236-9512. Creston C. Herold, Exec. Dir.

PURPOSE. To advance the professional growth of health-care personnel working in rehabilitation medicine.

MEMBERSHIP. *Requirements:* M.S. degree and three years experience in rehabilitation. *Dues:* based on annual income.

PUBLICATIONS. Periodicals. Payment required with order.

A44. AMERICAN CORRECTIVE THERAPY ASSOCIATION, INC., 1265 Cherry Rd., Memphis, Tenn. 38117. *Tel:* (901) 743-9312. Stanley H. Wertz, Exec. Dir.

PURPOSE. A professional association and one of the Allied Health Associations in the field of physical medicine and rehabilitation. *Specialization:* corrective therapy and remedial physical education.

MEMBERSHIP. *Requirements:* B.S. degree in physical education with special courses in adapted physical education and medical sciences.

PUBLICATIONS. Books, pamphlets, films, and periodicals. *Journal of Corrective Therapy*, $10/yr. Payment not required with order.

A45. AMERICAN COUNCIL ON ALCOHOL PROBLEMS, INC., 119 Constitution Ave. N.E., Washington, D.C. 20002. *Tel:* (202) 543-2441. William N. Plymat, Pres.

PURPOSE. To coordinate efforts of 40-state affiliated organizations in effort to reduce problems associated with use of alcohol. *Specialization:* addictive and dangerous substances.
PUBLICATIONS. Pamphlets on alcohol, alcoholism, marijuana; booklets on similar themes, plus LSD, venereal diseases, and cigarettes; Reader's Digest reprints. *The American Issue* (bimonthly). Emphasis on educational materials for schools. Payment required with order.

A46. AMERICAN   DENTAL   ASSOCIATION-BUREAU   OF   DENTAL HEALTH EDUCATION, 211 E. Chicago Ave., Chicago, Ill. 60611. *Tel:* (312) 944-6730. Dr. C. Gordon Watson, Exec. Dir.

PURPOSE. To encourage the improvement of health of the public and to promote the art and science of dentistry. *Specialization:* dental health.
PUBLICATIONS. Books, pamphlets, films, slides, records, and periodicals. Forty-page catalog of books and package libraries for dentists. Forty-five-page color-illustrated catalog of dental materials aimed at general public; posters and booklets on brushing and tooth care; handouts for dentists' offices; wall charts; and several dozen films and TV spots on dental care and oral hygiene. Abstracts for professionals. Payment required with order.

A47. AMERICAN DENTAL HYGIENISTS' ASSOCIATION, 211 E. Chicago Ave., Suite 1616, Chicago, Ill. 60611. *Tel:* (312) 944-7097. Carl H. Hauber, Exec. Dir.

PURPOSE. To improve oral health of the public and to advance art and science of dental hygiene.
MEMBERSHIP. *Requirements:* must be involved in dental hygiene. *Benefits:* most publications free to members.
PUBLICATIONS. *Dental Hygiene* (monthly) (through Charles B. Slack publishers); *Transactions* and *House of Delegates Manual*; career materials, manuals, and legislative information. Payment not required with order.

A48. AMERICAN DIABETES ASSOCIATION, 1 W. 48 St., New York, N.Y. 10020. *Tel:* (212) 541-4310. Ernest M. Frost, Exec. Vice-Pres.

PURPOSE. A voluntary health agency for education, detection, and research. *Specialization:* diabetes mellitus.
PUBLICATIONS. *Diabetes* (monthly); multivolume series on diagnosis and treatment of diabetes; meal-planning pamphlets (bulk rates available); patient education materials; *Diabetes Forecast* (bimonthly), for diabetics and their families; cookbooks; reprints. Payment required with order.

A49. AMERICAN FOUNDATION FOR THE BLIND, INC., 15 W. 16 St., New York, N.Y. 10011. *Tel:* (212) 924-0420. Loyal Eugene Apple, Exec. Dir.

PURPOSE. An agency for the improvement of welfare of the blind. *Specialization:* blindness.

SPECIAL INFORMATION SERVICES. *Special collections:* specialized library on blindness.

PUBLICATIONS. Books, pamphlets, films, and periodicals. Material free to public; nominal fees for professionals working in the field of service to the blind. Payment required with order except from institutions.

A50. AMERICAN GROUP PRACTICE ASSOCIATION, 20 S. Quaker Lane, Alexandria, Va. 22313. *Tel:* (703) 751-1000. James E. Cobb, Exec. Dir.

PURPOSE. To promote the growth and development of group practice. *Specialization:* group practice.

MEMBERSHIP. *Requirements:* legally organized bodies of three or more physicians practicing in a group and sharing resources. *Dues:* $500–$2,000/yr. *Benefits:* 50 percent discount on publication.

SPECIAL INFORMATION SERVICES. Placement Service, Group Practice Information Service, Consultation Service.

PUBLICATIONS. *Group Practice Journal* (bimonthly), compilation of articles of interest to group practitioners. Latest on malpractice, government involvement in health care, and activities of AGPA. Graphically exciting and well laid out. Also, one-page *Newsletter*; pamphlets on services offered by AGPA. Monographs on health-care delivery, funds for health-care organizations, topics related to HMO's, and setting up group practices. Payment required with order.

A51. AMERICAN GROUP PSYCHOTHERAPY ASSOCIATION, INC., 1865 Broadway, New York, N.Y. 10023. *Tel:* (212) 245-7732. Marsha Block, Admin. Sec.

PURPOSE. To provide information and to promote high standards in the field of group psychotherapy. *Specialization:* group psychotherapy.

MEMBERSHIP. *Requirements:* full members must be medical professionals with some experience in group therapy; associate members must have some experience in individual psychotherapy.

PUBLICATIONS. *International Journal of Group Psychotherapy* (quarterly); membership directory; *Suggested Guidelines for the Training of Group Therapists*; *History of AGPA*; *Consumers Guide to Group Psychotherapy*. Payment required with order.

A52. AMERICAN HEART ASSOCIATION, 44 E. 23 St., New York, N.Y. 10010.*

PURPOSE. To publish educational materials on heart diseases for the public and the medical profession. *Specialization:* research on the cardiovascular system and heart diseases.

PUBLICATIONS. Fifteen-page catalog of scientific journals and books that are aimed at physicians, investigators, and medical students. Journals listed include *Circulation* (monthly), devoted to clinical research and advances in cardiovascular field, $20/yr. in U.S.; *Circulation Research* (monthly) covers more basic research, $25/yr.; *Stroke—A Journal of Cerebral Circulation* (bimonthly), $25/yr.; *Recurring Bibliography of Hypertension* (bimonthly), $8/yr.; *Modern Concepts of Cardiovascular Disease* (monthly); *Cardiovascular Nursing* (bimonthly); *Current Concepts of Cerebrovascular Disease—Stroke* (quarterly). Also monographs, pamphlets (some free), results of symposia, reprints, and abstracts—all technical. Payment required with order.

A53. AMERICAN HOSPITAL ASSOCIATION, 840 N. Lake Shore Dr., Chicago, Ill. 60611. *Tel:* (312) 645-9400.

PURPOSE. To promote better public health through support of research, information, legislative lobbying, consultation, and public relations. *Specialization:* hospital administration and management.
MEMBERSHIP. *Requirements:* health-care institutions and individuals involved in hospital administration and management.
PUBLICATIONS. *Hospital Week, Washington Developments,* and *Trustee* (periodicals). Publications catalog lists dozens of books and pamphlets on hospital administration and public relations, ethics, inhalation therapy, nursing, statistics, chaplaincy, autopsies, dietary, and other areas of concern for managers of health-care institutions. Bulk rates available on some items. Payment required with individual order.

A54. AMERICAN INSTITUTE OF PHYSICS, 335 E. 45 St., New York, N.Y. 10017.*

PURPOSE. Publisher of journals and translator of foreign journals. *Specialization:* physics journals.
PUBLICATIONS.   Of interest to readers in field of health is *Physics in Medicine and Biology* (bimonthly), $73/yr. in U.S.; microfiche edition, $51/yr. Covers applications of theoretical and practical physics to medicine, physiology, and biology, including radiation dosimetry and related topics and instrumentation and computer applications. Includes extensive abstracts section in this field. Payment required with order.

A55. AMERICAN INSTITUTE OF THE HISTORY OF PHARMACY, Pharmacy Building, University of Wisconsin, Madison, Wis. 53706. *Tel:* (608) 262-4939. John Parascondola, Dir.

PURPOSE. An association to preserve, interpret, and promote the knowledge and appreciation of pharmacy's heritage. *Specialization:* history of pharmacology.
MEMBERSHIP. All interested persons. *Dues:* $15/yr. *Benefits:* members receive periodicals and a 40 percent discount on other publications.
SPECIAL INFORMATION SERVICES. Searches for material, photograph service, microfilms, photocopies. Answers queries on pharmaceutical history. Services mainly intended for members, scholars, and nonprofit institutions. *Special collections:* pharmacohistorical manuscript collection of Wisconsin State Historical Society; Audio-Visual History Collection; Drug Topics Photograph Collection.
PUBLICATIONS. Brochures describing pamphlets, slides, and periodicals (free). Booklets include guides to literature on pharmaceutical history; pamphlets describe antiques, numismatics, philately, and book collecting as they relate to pharmacy. Periodicals available are *Pharmacy in History* and *AIHP Notes.* Slide-talks, loaned to members without charge, include history of the drug jar, the drugstore, and quack therapy. Payment required with order.

A56. AMERICAN LIBRARY ASSOCIATION, 50 E. Huron St., Chicago, Ill. 60611.*

PURPOSE. A professional organization of librarians and libraries, publishing materials on library science, research, and other areas. *Specialization:* library science and communications.
PUBLICATIONS. Volumes of interest to health sciences librarians include *Bibliotherapy: Methods and Materials* (reading programs in group psychotherapy) and *Standards for Library Services in Health Care Institutions.* Many other titles on library science and communications sciences in 75-page catalog, including use and storage of audiovisual collections. Payment required with order of $5 or less.

A57. AMERICAN LUNG ASSOCIATION, 1740 Broadway, New York, N.Y. 10019. *Tel:* (202) CI 5-8000. Gerald R. Riso, Mng. Dir.

PURPOSE. To prevent and control respiratory diseases through education and community organization.
SPECIAL INFORMATION SERVICES. *Languages:* English and Spanish.
PUBLICATIONS. Fifteen-page catalog of selected publications. Includes books and booklets, leaflets, films, and posters on TB, asthma, air pollution, how to quit smoking, care of respiratory patients, flu, pleurisy, and other respiratory topics. Available journals are *American Review of Respiratory Disease, Basics of RD, ALA Bulletin,* and *Clinical Notes on Respiratory Diseases.* Fifteen films for general public, some with Spanish soundtrack. Two tape/slide self-teaching programs: *Measurement of Closing Volume* and *Interpretation of Blood Gases.* Computer tape program (in BASIC) on normal and abnormal lung function. Radio public service spots on records. Most items free. Payment not required with order.

A58. AMERICAN MEDICAL ASSOCIATION, Order Department, 535 N. Dearborn St., Chicago, Ill. 60610.*

PURPOSE. A professional organization of physicians promoting high standards of practice and publishing health education information for the public. *Specialization:* health education for physicians and the public.
SPECIAL INFORMATION SERVICES. *Languages:* English and Spanish.
PUBLICATIONS. List available from Order Department. Books and booklets for laymen and professionals, covering many topics: maternal and child care, physical education, statistics on health-care industry, human sexuality, scientific writing, peer review, and world nutrition. Results of symposia; advice on media relations. Pamphlets on alcohol, child care, advice for child readers, chronic and communicable diseases, doctor-patient relations, drugs, ecology, and mental health. Posters warning against smoking, alcohol, drugs, and venereal diseases. Many other materials on personal health care and fitness, plus record books for physicians. Payment required with order.

A59. AMERICAN MEDICAL RECORD ASSOCIATION, 875 N. Michigan Ave., Suite 1850, Chicago, Ill. 60611. *Tel:* (312) 787-2672. (Mrs.) Mary Waterstraat, RRA, Exec. Dir.

PURPOSE. "To promote the art and science of medical record administration." Members shall "strive to advance the knowledge and practice of medical record science, including continued self-improvement, in order to contribute to the best possible medical care."

MEMBERSHIP. *Requirements:* Accredited or registered medical record technicians and administrators. Those interested in the association may join as associates. Students in approved programs may join. *Dues:* $25–$40, depending on category; students $5.

SPECIAL INFORMATION SERVICES. The Foundation of Record Education Library at the AMRA headquarters welcomes requests. The Professional Services Division offers advice to members.

PUBLICATIONS. AMRA newsletter, *Counterpoint,* is published in alternate months from *Medical Record News* and is available only to members. *Medical Record News,* journal of the American Medical Record Association, is published bimonthly (February, April, June, August, October, December) and is free with membership or $12/yr. Cassette tapes of continuing education sessions (Recordfact series) are available for purchase. Payment required with publication order.

A60. AMERICAN MEDICAL STUDENT ASSOCIATION, 1400 Hicks Rd., Rolling Meadows, Ill. 60008. *Tel:* (312) 259-7450. Louis R. Giancola, Exec. Dir.

PURPOSE. An association to improve medical education and health-care delivery in the United States through the efforts of medical students. *Specialization:* medical education.

MEMBERSHIP. *Requirements:* medical students in U.S. medical schools. *Dues:* $5/4 yrs.

PUBLICATIONS. *New Physician* magazine, *Infusion* newsletter; pamphlets, films, and videotapes.

A61. AMERICAN MEDICAL TECHNOLOGISTS, 710 Higgins Rd., Park Ridge, Ill. 60068. *Tel:* (312) 823-5169. Chester B. Dziekonski, Exec. Sec.

PURPOSE. To certify credentials for medical laboratory personnel and to provide continuing education programs. *Specialization:* technical material for clinical laboratory personnel and information on careers in the field.

MEMBERSHIP. Members must meet educational and experiential requirements.

SPECIAL INFORMATION SERVICES. Career information.

PUBLICATIONS. *American Medical Technologists,* journal (bimonthly), with articles on research and techniques, new products, and news of the association, $5/yr. in U.S. Pamphlets on careers in medical technology, requirements for certification as medical assistant or technician, opportunities for ex-servicemen, AMT awards program. Payment not required with order.

A62. AMERICAN MEDICAL WOMEN'S ASSOCIATION, 1740 Broadway, New York, N.Y. 10019. *Tel:* (212) 586-8683. Lorraine Loesel, Exec. Dir.

PURPOSE. To promote interests common to women physicians. *Specialization:* women in medicine.

MEMBERSHIP. *Requirements:* M.D. degree.

PUBLICATIONS. *Journal of the American Medical Women's Association*, $15/yr.; career literature for women considering medicine as a career, $2.50. Payment required with order for career literature.

A63. AMERICAN NATURAL HYGIENE SOCIETY, INC., 1920 Irving Park Rd., Chicago, Ill. 60613. *Tel:* (312) 929-7420. Stanley L. Proror, Exec. Vice-Pres.

PURPOSE. To promote and educate the public in how to regain and maintain health through natural hygiene. *Specialization:* natural hygiene.
PUBLICATIONS. Books such as *Fasting for Renewal of Life, Hygienic Care of Children, Syphilis, The Werewolf of Medicine,* and *Fit Food for Man.* Publications stress raw foods, mental attitude, and fasting as ways to keep healthy. Periodical *Dr. Shelton's Hygienic Review* (monthly); informational pamphlets. Payment recommended with order.

A64. AMERICAN OCCUPATIONAL THERAPY ASSOCIATION, INC., 6000 Executive Blvd., Rockville, Md. 20852. *Tel:* (301) 770-2200. Gail S. Fidler, Interim Exec. Dir.

PURPOSE. Primarily a service organization for members and for students in occupational therapy; this association engages in consumer education and continuing education. *Specialization:* theory and practice of occupational therapy.
MEMBERSHIP. *Requirements:* occupational therapists with current dues paid.
PUBLICATIONS. Pamphlets, films, videotapes, and periodicals. A free catalog lists over 60 reprints from the *American Journal of Occupational Therapy* (35¢ each) and 11 reference works. Informational pamphlets are available in quantity. Audiovisual materials can be rented for three weeks or purchased (three 16mm films with sound and a resource manual for use in media approaches to promotion of occupational therapy). Payment required with order.

A65. AMERICAN OPTOMETRIC ASSOCIATION, 7000 Chippewa St., St. Louis, Mo. 63119. *Tel:* (314) 832-5770. J. Harold Bailey, Exec. Dir.

PURPOSE. To improve vision care and health of public and to promote art and science of optometric profession. *Specialization:* optometry.
PUBLICATIONS. Books, pamphlets, films, slides, and periodicals. *AOA News* and *AOA Journal.* Payment not required with order.

A66. AMERICAN ORTHOPSYCHIATRIC ASSOCIATION, INC., 1775 Broadway, New York, N.Y. 10019. *Tel:* (212) JU 6-5690.

PURPOSE. To promote collaborative approach to study and treatment of problems of human behavior. *Specialization:* orthopsychiatry.
MEMBERSHIP. *Requirements:* candidates must have endorsement from AOA members. *Dues:* $35/yr.; students $16/yr.
PUBLICATIONS. Books on motor gestalt tests. Set of 35mm slides on Bender test. *American Journal of Orthopsychiatry* (quarterly). Payment required with order.

A67. AMERICAN OSTEOPATHIC ASSOCIATION, 212 E. Ohio St., Chicago, Ill. 60611. *Tel:* (312) 944-2713. Edward P. Crowell, D.O., Exec. Dir.

PURPOSE. To promote health among the general public, encourage scientific research, and approve physician training programs in osteopathic institutions. *Specialization:* osteopathy.

MEMBERSHIP. *Requirements:* doctor of osteopathy degree.

PUBLICATIONS. Pamphlets on career outlook in osteopathic medicine, value of D.O. versus M.D. degree; promotion of wider acceptance and growth of teaching facilities, and legal, public relations, philosophic aspects of practice. *Journal of the AOA* for professional osteopaths (free to members); *D.O.* (monthly news); *Health* (bimonthly), a lay public health magazine; yearbook and directory of osteopathic physicians. Audiotapes for continuing education in medicine. Three films aimed at general audiences, no charge for loan except shipping costs. Payment required with order.

A68. AMERICAN PHARMACEUTICAL ASSOCIATION, 2215 Constitution Ave. N.W., Washington, D.C. 20037. *Tel:* (202) 628-4410. Dr. William S. Apple, Sec.

PURPOSE. An affiliation of professional pharmacists. *Specialization:* pharmacy and pharmaceuticals.

MEMBERSHIP. *Dues:* $55/yr.

PUBLICATIONS. Twelve-page publications catalog. Drug evaluations, dosage charts, handbooks, book reviews, and abstracts; *National Formulary. Journal of the American Pharmaceutical Association; APhA Weekly.* Films and slides. Payment required with order under $20.

INQUIRY ADDRESS. Publications Division, American Pharmaceutical Association, 2215 Constitution Ave. N.W., Washington, D.C. 20037. *Tel:* (202) 628-4410.

A69. AMERICAN PHYSICAL THERAPY ASSOCIATION, 1156 15 St. N.W., Washington, D.C. 20005. *Tel:* (202) 466-2070. Royce P. Noland, Exec. Dir.

PURPOSE. *Specialization:* physical therapy.

PUBLICATIONS. Books, pamphlets, and periodicals. Payment required with order.

A70. AMERICAN PHYSIOLOGICAL SOCIETY, c/o AV/MD, Stephen K. Herlitz, Inc., 850 Third Avenue, New York, N.Y. 10022.* *Tel:* (212) 421-6900. Orr E. Reynolds, Exec. Sec.

PURPOSE. A professional organization offering study programs to health professionals. *Specialization:* physiology.

PUBLICATIONS. Self-instructional slide-tape study programs. Eight lectures on renal physiology and six on cardiac. $45/lecture, $320 for Program I, $240 for Program II. Payment not required with order.

A71. AMERICAN PODIATRY ASSOCIATION, 20 Chevy Chase Circle, Washington, D.C. 20015. *Tel:* (202) 362-2700. Seward P. Nyman, D.P.M., Exec. Dir.

PURPOSE. An association for the promotion of the art and science of podiatry and the betterment of public health. *Specialization:* foot health.

MEMBERSHIP. *Requirements:* must be licensed podiatrist and member of state society. *Dues:* $175/yr.

PUBLICATIONS. Books, pamphlets, films, slides, records, and audiotapes on foot health. Pamphlets on topics such as foot health and aging, podiatry under Medicare, careers in the field, and foot care. Slides cover surgical techniques and diagnosis of foot problems; films cover same areas, plus public education and career guidance. Exhibits and posters. Catalog of instructional materials available. *Journal of the APA* (monthly). Payment required with order.

A72. AMERICAN PROFESSIONAL PRACTICE ASSOCIATION, 292 Madison Ave., New York, N.Y. 10017. *Tel:* (212) 949-5950. George Arden, Exec. Dir.

PURPOSE. To serve the business aspects of professional practice. *Specialization:* financial management.
MEMBERSHIP. *Requirements:* M.D., D.O., D.D.S., or D.M.D. degree or be a student studying for one of these degrees. *Dues:* $15/yr; students $7.50 (also includes interns, residents, and fellows). *Benefits:* financial counseling, practice management advice, and free publications.
PUBLICATIONS. *APPA Digest* (bimonthly), newsletter giving money management advice. *PC Update* (bimonthly) emphasizes professional corporations.

A73. AMERICAN PROTESTANT HOSPITAL ASSOCIATION, 840 N. Lake Shore Dr., Chicago, Ill. 60611. *Tel:* (312) 944-2814. Charles D. Phillips, Ed.D., Pres.

PURPOSE. A trade association of religiously affiliated hospitals and homes for the aged and a professional society for chaplains. *Specialization:* pastoral care, religious health-care delivery, and reports of convention proceedings.
PUBLICATIONS. *American Protestant Hospital Association Bulletin* available to members only. Audiotapes and pamphlets on pastoral care and religious health-care delivery available to general public. Payment not required with order.

A74. AMERICAN PSYCHIATRIC ASSOCIATION, 1700 18 St. N.W., Washington, D.C. 20009. *Tel:* (202) 232-7878. Melvin Sabshin, M.D., Medical Dir.

PURPOSE. A "society of medical specialists brought together by common interest in continuing study of psychiatry, in working together for more effective application of psychiatric knowledge . . . and in promoting mental health." *Specialization:* psychiatry.
MEMBERSHIP. *Requirements:* physician with some specialized training and experience in psychiatry.
PUBLICATIONS. Sixteen-page list. Dozens of books on mental illness, halfway houses, alcoholism, education, and behavior therapy. *American Journal of Psychiatry, Psychiatric News, Hospital and Community Psychiatry.* Also audiotapes. Payment not required with order.

A75. THE AMERICAN PSYCHOANALYTIC ASSOCIATION, One E. 57 St., New York, N.Y. 10022. *Tel:* (212) PL 2-0450. Helen Fischer, Admin. Dir.

PURPOSE. To study and advance psychoanalysis by advocating and maintaining standards for training and practice, fostering integration of the field with other branches of medicine, and encouraging research in all fields. *Specialization:* psychoanalysis.

MEMBERSHIP. *Requirements:* psychiatric resident or graduate of approved psychoanalytic training institute. *Dues:* $260/yr.

PUBLICATIONS. *Roster*, glossary of terms and concepts; *Freud Catalog*, summaries of papers from past meetings; *Journal of the American Psychoanalytic Association* (quarterly) (available from International Universities Press, 239 Park Ave. S., New York, N.Y. 10003), $20/yr; students $12. Payment required with order.

A76. AMERICAN PSYCHOLOGICAL ASSOCIATION, 1200 17 St. N.W., Washington, D.C. 20036. *Tel:* (202) 833-7600. C. Alan Boneau, Acting Exec. Off.

PURPOSE. To advance psychology as a science and as a means of promoting human welfare by encouragement of psychology in all its branches in the broadest and most liberal manner. *Specialization:* psychology.
MEMBERSHIP. Professional involvement or interest in psychology. *Dues:* $32–$47/yr.
PUBLICATIONS. Fifteen psychological journals and monthly newspaper. Subareas of psychology treated in individual journals include abnormal, applied, clinical, experimental, and comparative. Also abstracts, bulletin, Journal Supplement Abstract Service, and Employment Bulletin. Payment required with order.

A77. AMERICAN PUBLIC HEALTH ASSOCIATION, 1015 18 St. N.W., Washington, D.C. 20036.* *Tel:* (202) 467-5000. William H. McBeath, Exec. Dir.

PURPOSE. An association that "seeks to promote personal and environmental health."
PUBLICATIONS. *American Journal of Public Health* (monthly) and several other journals. Also monographs.

A78. AMERICAN SCHOOL HEALTH ASSOCIATION, Kent, Ohio 44240.*

PURPOSE. A professional organization concerned with the health of the school-age child. *Specialization:* health of the school-age child.
PUBLICATIONS. *Journal of School Health* (ten issues yearly). References for school nurses, curriculum guide in teaching about drugs, mental health in classroom, sex education for grades K–12, and bibliographies. Payment required with order.

A79. AMERICAN SOCIAL HEALTH ASSOCIATION, 1740 Broadway, New York, N.Y. 10019. *Tel:* (212) 582-3553. Donald P. Clough, Exec. Dir.

PURPOSE. To prevent, control, and eliminate sexually transmitted disease. *Specialization:* venereal disease.
MEMBERSHIP. *Dues:* $20/yr.
SPECIAL INFORMATION SERVICES. *Languages:* English and Spanish.
PUBLICATIONS. Pamphlets on the causes of venereal disease and its scope and extent in the United States, single copies free; bulk rates available. Payment not required with most orders.

A80. AMERICAN SOCIETY FOR ADOLESCENT PSYCHIATRY, 24 Green Valley Rd., Wallingford, Pa. 19086. *Tel:* (215) LO 6-1054. Julian I. Barish, M.D., Pres.

PURPOSE. To provide a national forum for psychiatrists interested in adolescents, to cooperate with other organizations in behalf of adolescents, and to facilitate communication and cooperation among constituent societies. *Specialization:* psychiatry of the adolescent.
MEMBERSHIP. *Requirements:* applicants join one of 16 local societies and automatically become national society members. Local societies limit membership to accredited psychiatrists; some locals open to allied professionals.
PUBLICATIONS. Newsletter (three a year); *Annals of Adolescent Psychiatry* (annual), $17.50; membership directory. Payment required with order.

A81. AMERICAN SOCIETY FOR CLINICAL PHARMACOLOGY AND THERAPEUTICS, 1718 Gallagher Rd., Norristown, Pa. 19401. *Tel:* (215) 277-3831. William B. Abrams, M.D., Pres.

PURPOSE. To promote and advance human pharmacology and therapeutics through support of research, education, and exchange of scientific information. (Services restricted to clinical pharmacologists and physicians concerned with therapeutics.) *Specialization:* clinical pharmacology.
MEMBERSHIP. *Requirements:* M.D. or Ph.D. degree in biomedical science or equivalent qualifications. Must demonstrate sincere interest in clinical pharmacology and therapeutics and have contributed to the literature.
PUBLICATIONS. *Clinical Pharmacology and Therapeutics* (monthly), free to members.

A82. AMERICAN SOCIETY FOR GASTROINTESTINAL ENDOSCOPY, 2799 W. Grand Blvd., Detroit, Mich. 48202. *Tel:* (313) 876-2408. Angelo E. Dagradi, Pres.

PURPOSE. To further knowledge of intestinal disease through the use of endoscopic instruments and to further teaching of gastrointestinal endoscopic methods of examination. *Specialization:* gastrointestinal endoscopy.
MEMBERSHIP. *Requirements:* physicians with special training and demonstrated skill in gastrointestinal endoscopy, who must be certified by specialty board. *Dues:* $50/yr.
PUBLICATIONS. *Gastrointestinal Endoscopy* (quarterly) (available from William S. Haubrich, M.D., ed., 476 Prospect Ave., La Jolla, Calif. 92037).

A83. AMERICAN SOCIETY FOR HOSPITAL PERSONNEL ADMINISTRATION, 840 N. Lake Shore Dr., Chicago, Ill. 60611. *Tel:* (312) 645-8253. Joseph Rosman, Sec.

PURPOSE. To provide educational resources and communication among members of hospital personnel management profession. (Services restricted to members.)
MEMBERSHIP. *Requirements:* must have personnel management responsibilities in a health-care institution.
PUBLICATIONS. Pamphlets, films, audio- and videotapes, and periodicals on personnel administration, labor relations, management development, supervisory training, and federal legislation affecting employment. Payment required with order.

A84. AMERICAN SOCIETY FOR MICROBIOLOGY, 1913 I St. N.W., Washington, D.C. 20006.*

PURPOSE. A professional organization for the advancement of microbiology. *Specialization:* microbiology.
MEMBERSHIP. *Requirements:* B.S. degree in microbiology or related field or equivalent training and experience. *Dues:* from $20. *Benefits:* newsletter and one of journals listed below; special rates on additional subscriptions and other publications.
PUBLICATIONS. Books on Proceedings of Fifth International Spore Conference held in Fontana, Wisconsin ("Spore V"), numerical taxonomy, clinical microbiology techniques, antimicrobial agents, and chemotherapy. Journals include *Antimicrobial Agents and Chemotherapy* (monthly), *Journal of Bacteriology* (monthly), *Applied Microbiology* (monthly), *Bacteriological Reviews* (quarterly), *Journal of Virology* (monthly), *Infection and Immunity* (monthly), and *International Journal of Systematic Bacteriology* (quarterly). Also monthly newsletter of ASM, abstracts, and membership directory. Payment not required with order.

A85. AMERICAN SOCIETY FOR PHARMACOLOGY AND EXPERIMENTAL THERAPEUTICS, INC., 9650 Rockville Pike, Bethesda, Md. 20014. *Tel:* (301) 530-7060. Dr. Ellisworth B. Cook, Exec. Off.

PURPOSE. To promote pharmacological knowledge and its application and to conduct research in that field. *Specialization:* pharmacology, clinical pharmacology, and drug metabolism.
MEMBERSHIP. *Requirements:* qualified investigators with achievements in research in pharmacology.
PUBLICATIONS. Pamphlets and periodicals.

A86. AMERICAN SOCIETY FOR TESTING AND MATERIALS, 1916 Race St., Philadelphia, Pa. 19103.*

PURPOSE. To test and develop standards for building materials, scientific instruments, chemicals, and other products used in science and industry. *Specialization:* developing technical standards and testing materials.
PUBLICATIONS. Thirty-page catalog of publications lists books of standards and data on several hundred different substances. Includes nine volumes in radiology, several on X-ray technology, and some in mass spectrometry that may be of help to lab technicians and researchers using advanced procedures. *Journal of Forensic Sciences* (quarterly) carries papers on instrumental analysis, pathology, and other areas, $33/yr; members $22/yr. Payment required with journal order and with order under $6 for other materials.

A87. AMERICAN SOCIETY OF ABDOMINAL SURGEONS, 675 Main St., Melrose, Mass. 02176. *Tel:* (617) 665-6102. Blaise F. Alfano, M.D., Exec. Sec.

PURPOSE. To advocate continuing education for abdominal surgeons. *Specialization:* abdominal surgery.
PUBLICATIONS. *Journal of Abdominal Surgery*, texts, and slide-sound programs. Payment required with order.

A88. AMERICAN SOCIETY OF ALLIED HEALTH PROFESSIONS, One DuPont Circle, Suite 300, Washington, D.C. 20036. *Tel:* (202) 293-3422. William M. Samuels, Exec. Dir.

PURPOSE. To promote high standards in education and utilization of persons in allied health professions. *Specialization:* allied health professions.
MEMBERSHIP. Open to institutions (primarily schools preparing health professionals), allied health educators and practitioners and others with strong interest in field, and companies. *Dues:* $25–$1,000/yr.
SPECIAL INFORMATION SERVICES. Studies on core curricula, accreditation, and health careers counseling.
PUBLICATIONS. Newsletter *Allied Health Trends* (monthly); *Journal of Allied Health* (quarterly); "Institutional Update" (monthly) sent to institutional members. Payment not required with order.

A89. AMERICAN SOCIETY OF CLINICAL PATHOLOGISTS, INC., 2100 W. Harrison St., Chicago, Ill. 60612. *Tel:* (312) 738-1336. David L. Gilcrest, Exec. Dir.

PURPOSE. To serve pathologists and laboratory medicine professionals by producing continuing medical education materials and workshops. *Specialization:* laboratory medicine.
MEMBERSHIP. *Requirements:* pathologist, pathology resident, other physician or Ph.D., medical technologist, or other laboratory specialist. *Dues:* vary. *Benefits:* members receive two journals and 20 percent discount on publications.
SPECIAL INFORMATION SERVICES. National, regional, and local workshops.
PUBLICATIONS. Twenty-page materials catalog. Slides, tape cassettes, and audiovisual programs on anatomic pathology and lab techniques. Slide sets and atlases, lab manuals, self-assessment programs, subscription materials, and summary reports. Ten rental films on lab technique, anatomy, and blood banks. "Professional Education" series will eventually number 36 programs on videocassettes. *American Journal of Clinical Pathology*, *Laboratory Medicine*, and *ASCP Newsletter*.

A90. AMERICAN SOCIETY OF HEMATOLOGY, National Slide Bank, University of Washington, Seattle, Wash. 98195.*

PURPOSE. To provide slides to physicians. *Specialization:* hematology.
PUBLICATIONS. Brochure lists slides (also available as microfiche) by category, as well as audiotape/slide teaching sets. Twenty-one of latter on blood morphology, hemophilia, and hemostasis. Payment not required with order.

A91. AMERICAN SOCIETY OF HOSPITAL ATTORNEYS, 840 N. Lake Shore Dr., Chicago, Ill. 60611, *Tel:* (312) 645-8210. William F. Steigman, Acting Sec.

PURPOSE. To educate, disseminate to, and share information with attorneys representing hospitals, in particular, and active in medical-legal field, generally. (Services restricted to members of the society and hospital members of AHA.) *Specialization:* hospital laws.
MEMBERSHIP. *Requirements:* attorney who represents hospitals that are members of the American Hospital Association. *Dues:* $35–$60.

SPECIAL INFORMATION SERVICES. Compendium of information and files in field of hospital law.
PUBLICATIONS. Periodicals and other publications. Available to members only.
INQUIRY ADDRESS. American Society of Hospital Attorneys, 840 N. Lake Shore Dr., Chicago, Ill. *Tel:* (312) 645-8226.

A92. AMERICAN SOCIETY OF HOSPITAL PHARMACISTS, 4630 Montgomery Ave., Washington, D.C. 20014. *Tel:* (301) 657-3000. Joseph A. Oddis, Exec. Dir.

PURPOSE. A national specialty society of pharmacists engaged in institutional practice of pharmacy. *Specialization:* professional practice of pharmacy and drug information.
MEMBERSHIP. *Requirements:* practicing or studying institutional pharmacy or retired from field.
PUBLICATIONS. *American Journal of Hospital Pharmacy* (monthly); *ASHP Newsletter* (monthly); *Voices 12/60* (monthly), cassette tape program; *Formulary Service*, drug information subscription service. Also books, pamphlets, slide-tape programs, and reprints. Payment required with order under $20.

A93. AMERICAN SOCIETY OF INTERNAL MEDICINE, 703 Market St., Suite 535, San Francisco, Calif. 94103. *Tel:* (415) 777-1000. William R. Ramsey, Exec. Dir.

PURPOSE. To study scientific, economic, social, and political aspects of medicine to secure good patient care and high standards of practice in internal medicine. *Specialization:* internal medicine.
MEMBERSHIP. *Requirements:* three years AMA-approved training in internal medicine plus two years additional experience in internal medicine. *Dues:* $80/yr.
PUBLICATIONS. Brochures for practice (diagnosis forms, questionnaires, personal history, flow sheets), waiting rooms (patient information), and on group insurance and business affairs. Bulk rates, free single samples. Also periodicals. Payment required with order.

A94. AMERICAN SOCIETY OF TROPICAL MEDICINE AND HYGIENE, Box 15208, Druid Hills Br., Atlanta, Ga. 30333. *Tel:* (404) 633-3311. George R. Healy, Sec.-Treas.

PURPOSE. To advance tropical medicine and hygiene, including medicine, nursing, engineering, entomology, parasitology, and allied specialties in this field.
MEMBERSHIP. Interest in any phase of tropical medicine and hygiene, including all arthropod-borne diseases, medical care, and human welfare. *Dues:* $15/yr.
PUBLICATIONS. *American Journal of Tropical Medicine and Hygiene* and *Tropical Medicine and Hygiene News.*

A95. AMERICAN SOCIOLOGICAL ASSOCIATION, 1722 N St. N.W., Washington, D.C. 20036. *Tel:* (202) 833-3410. Otto N. Larsen, Exec. Off.

PURPOSE. To disseminate sociological knowledge. *Specialization:* sociology.
MEMBERSHIP. Open to persons interested in or studying sociology.
PUBLICATIONS. *Journal of Health and Social Behavior* (quarterly), covering aspects of social life bearing on human health. Payment required with order.

A96. AMERICAN THORACIC SOCIETY, 1740 Broadway, New York, N.Y. 10019. *Tel:* (212) 245-8000. R. Weymueller, Exec. Dir.

PURPOSE. To promote control and prevention of lung disease.
MEMBERSHIP. *Requirements:* M.D., R.N., or allied health professions with interest in respiratory diseases. *Dues:* $32.
PUBLICATIONS. Books, pamphlets, films, slides, audiotapes, and periodicals. Payment required with some orders.

A97. AMERICAN VETERINARY MEDICAL ASSOCIATION, Film Library, 600 S. Michigan Ave., Chicago, Ill. 60605.* *Tel:* (312) 922-7930.

PURPOSE. A professional organization providing free-loan 16mm films for continuing education of veterinarians and for public showings. *Specialization:* veterinary medicine.
PUBLICATIONS. Eighteen-page brochure of films of general interest and of technical subjects, produced by USDA, state agencies, farmers' groups, and others. Large selection for veterinary teaching programs. Payment not required with order; $5 fee required from nonmembers.

A98. THE ARTHRITIS FOUNDATION, 475 Riverside Dr., New York, N.Y. 10027. *Tel:* (212) 678-6363. Charles B. Harding, Chmn. of the Board.

PURPOSE. To seek the cause, prevention, and cure for arthritis; to help arthritis sufferers; to train scientists and physicians; and to support research. Seventy-four local chapters. *Specialization:* rheumatic diseases.
SPECIAL INFORMATION SERVICES. Local referrals to medical care services and aid.
PUBLICATIONS. *Arthritis and Rheumatism* (six issues per year) and *Bulletin on Rheumatic Diseases* (nine issues per year). Professional-oriented manuals, monographs, and films for physicians, covering arthritis and rheumatism. Literature for patients and the public includes pamphlets, handbooks, leaflets, and reprints. Slide series for health-care personnel. Payment required with order.

A99. ASSOCIATION FOR THE ADVANCEMENT OF BEHAVIOR THERAPY, 475 Park Ave. S., New York, N.Y. 10016. *Tel:* (212) 889-0721. Richard B. Stuart, Pres.

PURPOSE. To promote general advancement of theory and techniques underlying various facets of behavior therapy. *Specialization:* behavior therapy.
MEMBERSHIP. Open to individuals who are professionals in pertinent fields of behavior therapy. *Dues:* $10–20.
PUBLICATIONS. *Behavior Therapy* (five issues per year).

A100. ASSOCIATION FOR THE ADVANCEMENT OF HEALTH EDUCATION, 1201 16 St. N.W., Washington, D.C. 20036. *Tel:* (202) 833-5535. John H. Cooper, Exec. Sec.

PURPOSE. To advance health education. *Specialization:* health education.
MEMBERSHIP. Individuals in schools, universities, health and education administration, and public and private health services.

PUBLICATIONS. List available. Books and leaflets in athletics, dance, fitness, research, and safety education. Abstracts and bibliographies of research papers. Films and filmstrips on sex education, drug abuse, and physical education. Payment not required with institutional order.

A101. ASSOCIATION FOR THE STUDY OF ABORTION, 120 W. 57 St., New York, N.Y. 10021. *Tel:* (212) 245-2360. Jimmye Kimmey, Exec. Dir.

PURPOSE. To educate and provide information in the field of abortion rights. *Specialization:* abortion.
MEMBERSHIP. Names added to mailing list on request.
PUBLICATIONS. Reprints of articles and legal cases and judicial opinions. Several dozen publications, plus newsletter. Film, *An Unfinished Story*, tells of woman facing decision on abortion; free rental. Most materials free; contributions asked for some.

A102. ASSOCIATION OF AMERICAN MEDICAL COLLEGES, One DuPont Circle N.W., Washington, D.C. 20036. *Tel:* (202) 466-5100. John A. D. Cooper, M.D., Pres.

PURPOSE. An association organized to carry out purposes and operate for benefit of member institutions—medical schools of nonprofit educational institutions and nonprofit teaching hospitals. *Specialization:* medical education.
MEMBERSHIP. *Dues:* individuals $20/yr.; medical students $10/yr.
PUBLICATIONS. *Journal of Medical Education* (monthly), free to members; directories to member institutions; medical school admissions; *AAMC Bulletin* (monthly), newsletter. Catalog of publications lists dozens of works on minorities in medicine, physician performance measurement, salaries, curricula, and periodicals on medical education. Various divisions of association (Biomedical Research, Teaching Hospitals, etc.) produce publications in their particular fields. Payment required with order.

A103. ASSOCIATION OF MENTAL HEALTH ADMINISTRATORS, 2901 Lafayette, Lansing, Mich. 48906. *Tel:* (517) 484-2896. James C. Hodges, Exec. Dir.

PURPOSE. To promote better administration in health-care delivery systems. *Specialization:* mental health administration.
MEMBERSHIP. Mental health-care organizations and individuals engaged in administration of treatment/care services. *Dues:* organizations $50–$300, depending on size of budget.
PUBLICATIONS. *Journal of Mental Health Administration*, nonmembers $10/yr.; newsletter (bimonthly), except for libraries not available to nonmembers; topical monographs and papers. Payment required with nonmember order.

A104. ASSOCIATION OF MILITARY SURGEONS OF THE UNITED STATES, 8502 Connecticut Ave., Chevy Chase, Md. 20015. *Tel:* (301) 657-1980.

PURPOSE. *Specialization:* military medicine.
PUBLICATIONS. *Military Medicine* (monthly), journal of the Society of the Federal Medical Agencies, $20/yr. in U.S.

A105. ASSOCIATION OF OPERATING ROOM NURSES, 10170 E. Mississippi Ave., Denver, Colo. 80231. *Tel:* (303) 755-6300. Ms. Jerry G. Peers, Exec. Dir.

PURPOSE. A professional organization of registered nurses in charge of or associated with operating rooms. *Specialization:* operating room nursing.
MEMBERSHIP. Must be registered professional nurse engaged in operating room nursing.
SPECIAL INFORMATION SERVICES. Nursing education and continuing education information available from Education Department.
PUBLICATIONS. *AORN Journal* (monthly); reprints of past articles available. Brochures on careers in operating room nursing; educational programs guide; historical and informational brochures on AORN. List of films on nursing distributed by American College of Surgeons Surgical Film Library/Davis and Geck. Payment required with order.

A106. THE ATHLETIC INSTITUTE, 705 Merchandise Mart, Chicago, Ill. 60654. *Tel:* (312) 644-3020. Don Bushore, Exec. Dir.

PURPOSE. A nonprofit organization devoted to advancement of athletics, physical education, and recreation. *Specialization:* sports and physical education.
SPECIAL INFORMATION SERVICES. Free *Sources of Official Rules*, listings for most sports.
PUBLICATIONS. Distributes official rules books for many sports. Thirty-page catalog of audiovisual and published instructional aids; *Sports Techniques*, series of books; books for professional instructors of sport; film loops and videotapes on preventing injuries. Informational brochure on services of institute. Payment required with order under $10.

A107. BIOMEDICAL ENGINEERING SOCIETY, Box 2399, Culver City, Calif. 90230. *Tel:* (000) 789-3811. Ernst Attinger, Pres.

PURPOSE. To encourage development, dissemination, integration, and utilization of knowledge in biomedical engineering. *Specialization:* biomedical engineering.
MEMBERSHIP. *Requirements:* must be distinguished or active in biomedical engineering or a student in the field. *Dues:* full or associate member $10; student $5.
PUBLICATIONS. *Annals of Biomedical Engineering* (quarterly) (nonmembers order from Academic Press, 111 Fifth Ave., New York, N.Y.). Also directory and informational brochures.

A108. CALIFORNIA PEACE OFFICERS' ASSOCIATION, 800 Forum Building, Sacramento, Calif. 95814. *Tel:* (916) 446-7847. John F. Duffy, Pres.

PURPOSE. A professional organization of California law enforcement officials. *Specialization:* law enforcement and public safety.
MEMBERSHIP. *Requirements:* open to law enforcement officials and judicial personnel in California, as well as legislators and persons involved in private security in California. *Dues:* $10–$20/yr.
PUBLICATIONS. *Journal of California Law Enforcement* (quarterly) includes articles on public safety and health and welfare of peace officers in terms of legal responsibil-

ity. Films on handling mentally ill suspects, effects of marijuana, and emergency childbirth. Payment not required with order.

A109. CANCER CARE, INC. and THE NATIONAL CANCER FOUNDATION, INC., One Park Ave., New York, N.Y. 10016. *Tel:* (212) 679-5700. Irene G. Buckley, Exec. Dir.

PURPOSE. To provide direct services for advanced cancer patients and their families in tristate, 50-mile radius area around and including New York City. *Specialization:* service for advanced cancer patients and their families.
MEMBERSHIP. Seventy-eight local chapters throughout the area served. *Dues:* none.
PUBLICATIONS. Annual reports and results of symposia. Emphasis on financing and providing care during catastrophic illnesses, advanced cancer in particular. Films on cancer care and coping with a member of the family with advanced cancer. Cancer information available both inside and outside 50-mile radius of direct service. Payment not required with order.

A110. THE CARR FOUNDATION, 10350 Wyton Dr., Los Angeles, Calif. 90024. *Tel:* (213) 276-2676. Omar John Fareed, M.D., Pres. and Medical Dir.

PURPOSE. To deal with nutrition, overpopulation, and world communication.

A111. CEREAL INSTITUTE, INC., 135 S. LaSalle St., Chicago, Ill. 60603.* *Tel:* (312) 782-7140. Eugene B. Hayden, Pres.

PURPOSE. An organization promoting benefits and nutritive value of American breakfast cereals. *Specialization:* breakfast cereals.
PUBLICATIONS. Information on nutrition, emphasizing the American breakfast cereals as an integral part of today's affluent, rakish lifestyles. Cereals resource kit, *Breakfast Cereals in Today's Lifestyle*, for morning grain-munchers young and old. Consists of sound-filmstrip with booklet.

A112. CHILD WELFARE LEAGUE OF AMERICA, INC., 67 Irving Place, New York, N.Y. 10003.*

PURPOSE. "Voluntary membership organization with accrediting, standard-setting, research, legislative, library and information functions." *Specialization:* child welfare.
PUBLICATIONS. Catalog lists over 100 titles, ranging from 25¢ pamphlets to books at about $10. Topics covered include day care, adoption, sex education, mental health, child abuse, and standards for family services. *Child Welfare*, journal, $8/yr. Payment required with order from individuals. Institutions are billed for order over $10. Bulk rate available. Address orders to Publications Order Department.

A113. CHILDBIRTH WITHOUT PAIN EDUCATION ASSOCIATION, 20134 Snowden, Detroit, Mich. 48235. *Tel:* (313) 341-3816. Flora Hommel, Exec. Dir.

PURPOSE. To teach preparation for childbirth through the psychoprophylactic, or Lamaze, method of painless childbirth; to train instructors and monitrices (labor coaches); and to provide the public with related information. *Specialization:* painless childbirth through Lamaze-Pavlov method.

MEMBERSHIP. *Dues:* individual \$2.50/yr.; higher rates for professionals. *Benefits:* voting privileges and newsletter.

SPECIAL INFORMATION SERVICES. Materials for professionals on childbirth education.

PUBLICATIONS. Brochure "Childbirth Can Be Painless and Joyful"; film *American Naissance: Journey with a Friend*; newsletter (monthly).

A114. COLLEGE OF AMERICAN PATHOLOGISTS, 7400 N. Skokie Blvd., Skokie, Ill. 60076. *Tel:* (312) 677-3500. Howard E. Cartwright, Exec. Dir.

PURPOSE. To foster high standards in pathology, to advance the science of pathology, and to improve medical laboratory service.

MEMBERSHIP. *Requirements:* must be certified by American Board of Pathology or equivalent.

PUBLICATIONS. List of publications, many of which are on subscription basis, includes educational programs, evaluation services, and self-study programs. Periodicals include *Inspection and Accreditation Newsletter*, *Legislative Keyhole*, *Q Tips*, and others. Books on aerospace pathology, lab regulations and maintenance, and handling specimens. Also slide/sound packages.

A115. THE COMMONWEALTH FUND, One E. 75 St., New York, N.Y. 10021. *Tel:* (212) 535-0400. Carleton B. Chapman, M.D., Pres.

PURPOSE. To support innovative developments in medical education and certain aspects of the health-care system. (Services, awarding of grants, restricted to medical schools and established health-care organizations.)

PUBLICATIONS. Publishes books through Harvard University Press to which orders are sent. Annual reports on fund activities.

A116. CONVENTION OF AMERICAN INSTRUCTORS OF THE DEAF, INC., 5034 Wisconsin Ave. N.W., Washington, D.C. 20016. *Tel:* (202) 363-1327. Howard M. Quigley, Exec. Dir.

PURPOSE. To serve and unite all persons actively and directly engaged in the education of the deaf. *Specialization:* education of the deaf.

MEMBERSHIP. Must be actively and directly engaged in, or preparing students to enter, field of deaf education. Students may also join. *Dues:* \$15/yr.; students \$10/yr. *Benefits:* subscription to journal.

PUBLICATIONS. Proceedings of biennial meetings; *American Annals of the Deaf* (six issues per year), oldest educational periodical in the United States, begun in 1847. Payment required with order.

A117. THE COUNCIL FOR EXCEPTIONAL CHILDREN, 1920 Association Dr., Reston, Va. 22091. *Tel:* (703) 620-3660. William C. Geer, Exec. Dir.

PURPOSE. To promote the advancement and education of all exceptional children. (Services restricted to students, special education teachers, administrators, and others involved in studying or teaching exceptional children.) *Specialization:* handicapped children, learning disabilities, health impairments, and mental retardation.

MEMBERSHIP. All persons concerned with education of exceptional children. *Dues:* \$25/yr. *Benefits:* members receive three periodicals.

SPECIAL INFORMATION SERVICES. Custom computer searches at toll-free number (800) 336-3728, topical bibliographies, and special publications.

PUBLICATIONS. *Exceptional Children* (eight issues per year); *Teaching Exceptional Children* (quarterly); *Update* (six issues per year); topical bibliographies; education abstracts; books, audiocassettes, manuals, and research papers on learning disabilities, aural handicaps, dyslexia, therapy, autism, child abuse, status of laws, and gifted children. Large and comprehensive selections. Payment required with order under $25.

INQUIRY ADDRESS. CEC Information Services, 1920 Association Dr., Reston, Va. 22091.

A118. COUNCIL OF PLANNING LIBRARIANS EXCHANGE BIBLIOGRAPHIES, Box 229, Monticello, Ill. 61856. *Tel:* (217) 762-3831. Mary Vance, Ed.

PURPOSE. A nationally organized group of librarians, faculty, professional planners, public and private planning organizations, and others interested in problems of library organization and research and the dissemination of information on city and regional planning. *Specialization:* bibliographies in planning and public health.

PUBLICATIONS. Compiled bibliographies can be subscribed to for 40 consecutive issues. Bibliographies cited concentrate on urban planning, but health planning, health-care delivery systems, community facilities, careers, aging and the aged, maternal care, and other topics are listed. Payment not required with order.

A119. THE DEVEREUX FOUNDATION, 19 S. Waterloo Rd., Devon, Pa. 19333. *Tel:* (215) 687-3000. Marshall H. Jarvis, Pres.

PURPOSE. A national network of residential and day facilities for treatment, education, and rehabilitation of emotionally disturbed and mentally impaired children, adolescents, and young adults. (Services restricted to mental health workers and educators.) *Specialization:* motor achievement measurement and therapy.

PUBLICATIONS. Films on IMAGE (individual motor achievement through guided education) for general public and professional audiences. This is a method for measuring child's level of motor functioning and creating individual exercise program. Two 16mm color films for rent. Manuals for professionals on rating behavior in children and adolescents. IMAGE kit containing graphs, tests, and materials for pinpointing motor difficulties in children and designing therapy exercises. Catalog for professionals available. Payment required with order.

A120. DRUG ABUSE COUNCIL, 1828 L St. N.W., Washington, D.C. 20036.*

PURPOSE. "To serve on a national level as an independent source of needed research, public policy evaluation, and program guidance in the areas of drug use and misuse." *Specialization:* drug abuse.

SPECIAL INFORMATION SERVICES. A library and information center are available to researchers, students, workers in the field, and the general public.

PUBLICATIONS. A number of series are produced and available at little or no charge, including: Public Policy series (free), Monograph series, Handbook series, Fellows series, and Special Studies series. Payment required with order.

A121. DRUG, CHEMICAL AND ALLIED TRADES ASSOCIATION, 350 Fifth Ave., Suite 3014, New York, N.Y. 10001. *Tel:* (212) 736-8884. Joseph D. Madden, Exec. Vice-Pres.

PURPOSE. A forum for the exchange of useful information and promotion of business contacts for members. *Specialization:* chemical and drug trades.
MEMBERSHIP. *Requirements:* open to firms, not individuals.
PUBLICATIONS. Biweekly digest of current activities and trends, for members only.

A122. THE EDUCATIONAL FOUNDATION OF THE AMERICAN SOCIETY OF PLASTIC AND RECONSTRUCTIVE SURGEONS, INC., 29 E. Madison Ave., Suite 807, Chicago, Ill. 60602. *Tel:* (312) 641-0593. William C. Grabb, M.D., Pres.

PURPOSE. The education of plastic surgeons. *Specialization:* plastic surgery.
MEMBERSHIP. *Requirements:* board certification in plastic surgery. *Dues:* voluntary contributions.
PUBLICATIONS. Films, slides, and videotapes. Also instructional booklets for undergraduate medical students. Payment not required with order.

A123. EMPHYSEMA ANONYMOUS, INC., 1364 Palmetto Ave., Box 66, Fort Myers, Fla. 33902. *Tel:* (813) 334-4226. Jennie Winch Barkus, Natl. Pres.

PURPOSE. A volunteer organization dedicated to helping emphysema victims toward a more useful life by means of education, encouragement, and mutual assistance. *Specialization:* emphysema.
PUBLICATIONS. Brochures on organization's history; "Teaching the Patient to Help Himself" and "Our Daily Breath" with spiritual and physical exercises; bimonthly newsletter *Batting the Breeze.* Emphasis in publications on spiritual uplifting and mental attitude. Payment not required with order.

A124. EPILEPSY FOUNDATION OF AMERICA, 1828 L St. N.W., Suite 406, Washington, D.C. 20036.* Peter Van Haverbeke, Mgr., Broadcast and Audiovisual Department.

PURPOSE. An organization devoted to research on epilepsy, offering audiovisual materials on the disease to the public. *Specialization:* epilepsy.
PUBLICATIONS. About ten films available for purchase or loan (latter costs only small service charge). Contact regional office in Boston, Atlanta, Chicago, Houston, or Los Angeles for further details.

A125. EUTHANASIA EDUCATIONAL COUNCIL, 250 W. 57 St., New York, N.Y. 10019. *Tel:* (212) 246-6962. Elizabeth T. Halsey, Exec. Dir.

PURPOSE. An educational nonprofit organization devoted to establishing the right to die with dignity. *Specialization:* educational materials on euthanasia.
MEMBERSHIP. *Requirement:* minimum contribution of $3.
PUBLICATIONS. *Euthanasia News* (monthly) newsletter; pamphlets on medical, legal, social, and ethical aspects of euthanasia; proceedings of recent conferences; case histories; a patient Bill of Rights and a Living Will, by which one can request

euthanasia in event of loss of faculties. Free literature on request; contributions encouraged.

A126. FAMILY SERVICE ASSOCIATION OF AMERICA, 44 E. 23 St., New York, N.Y. 10010.*

PURPOSE. *Specialization:* family services.
PUBLICATIONS. About 75 titles are listed in catalog. Some are pamphlets and some books. Most are geared toward the professional working with families, but some are for families themselves. Topics include administration, casework theory, children, ethnic groups, the family, illegitimacy, and research. Payment required for order from individuals; institutions may be billed for order over $10.

A127. GASP (GROUP AGAINST SMOG AND POLLUTION), Box 5165, Pittsburgh, Pa. 15206. *Tel:* (412) 441-6650. Arthur R. Gorr, Pres.

PURPOSE. To clean up and enhance the environment through prevention of land, air, and water pollution. *Specialization:* pollution and its elimination.
MEMBERSHIP. Interest and payment of dues.
Special INFORMATION SERVICES. Speakers, action on complaints, and lawyer referral.
PUBLICATIONS. *Hotline* (newsletter), Action bulletins, technical reports, fund-raiser cookbooks, and informational pamphlets. Much of local interest to Allegheny County, Pa., residents, but general information on pollution also supplied. Film on effects of steelmills' pollution in Pittsburgh for rent or sale. Payment required with order.

A128. GERONTOLOGICAL SOCIETY, One DuPont Circle, Suite 520, Washington, D.C. 20036. *Tel:* (202) 659-4698. Edwin Kaskowitz, Exec. Dir.

PURPOSE. A professional organization devoted to research, education, and practice in field of aging. *Specialization:* gerontology.
MEMBERSHIP. *Requirements:* professional or graduate student in field of aging. *Dues:* $35/yr. *Benefits:* subscription to two journals.
PUBLICATIONS. *Journal of Gerontology* and *The Gerontologist* (both six issues per year). A few books on research and practice in gerontology.

A129. THE GILLES DE LA TOURETTE SYNDROME ASSOCIATION, Bell Plaza Building, 42–40 Bell Blvd., Bayside, N.Y. 11361.*

PURPOSE. An organization of those afflicted with Tourette syndrome (disorder of the central nervous system believed to be an organic dysfunction, exact cause still unknown), as well as their relatives and others who are interested. Aids patients, publishes medical and nonmedical information, and raises funds for research. *Specialization:* Gilles de la Tourette syndrome.
PUBLICATIONS. Newsletter, pamphlet "A Guide for Patients," and other information on Tourette syndrome. Information free; contributions welcomed.

GROUP AGAINST SMOG AND POLLUTION *See* A127

A130. GROUP FOR THE ADVANCEMENT OF PSYCHIATRY, Publications Office, 419 Park Ave. S., New York, N.Y. 10016. *Tel:* (212) 889-5760. Judd Marmor, Pres.

PURPOSE. To collect and appraise significant data in psychiatry, mental health, and human relations and to apply this knowledge for promotion of mental health and good human relations. *Specialization:* psychiatry.
PUBLICATIONS. Thirty-page catalog of reports and symposia. Offerings are findings by some 21 working committees formed from the group's 300 members, and cover aging, childhood, law, medical education, psychopathology, social issues, therapy, as well as other topics. Also bound collections of GAP publications for use in offices and libraries. Payment required with order under $5.

A131. HAY FEVER PREVENTION SOCIETY, INC. and/or FORD, STERN, JACKSON MEMORIAL LIBRARY, 2300 Sedgwick Ave., Suite 2-G, Bronx, N.Y. 10468. *Tel:* (212) 295-1069.

PURPOSE. To eradicate ragweed and to provide information on ragweed hay fever to schools and libraries. *Specialization:* ragweed.
MEMBERSHIP. *Dues:* $6/yr.
PUBLICATIONS. Pamphlets warning "Get ragweed before it gets you!" Organization urges national program to chemically eradicate these plants to alleviate hay fever misery. Distributes pamphlet printed by Dow Chemical Co. promoting large-scale application of 2,4-dichlorophenoxyacetic acid. Token charge for printed matter. Books loaned on deposit. Payment not required with order.

A132. HEALTH SCIENCES COMMUNICATIONS ASSOCIATION (HESCA), Box 79, Millbrae, Calif. 94030. *Tel:* (415) 666-1958. Thomas L. Banks, Assoc. Mgr.

PURPOSE. To extend health sciences education and communication.
MEMBERSHIP. *Dues:* $40/yr.
PUBLICATIONS. *Journal of Biocommunications;* newsletter, free to members; individuals and libraries $17.50/yr.; students $12/yr. Payment required with order.

A133. THE HOGG FOUNDATION FOR MENTAL HEALTH, University of Texas, Austin, Tex. 78712. *Tel:* (512) 471-5041.

PURPOSE. To fund programs and publish materials emphasizing positive aspects of mental health. *Specialization:* mental health.
PUBLICATIONS. Thirty-page list covering materials on mental health from childhood to old age; for the most part, they are nontechnical and aimed at the general public. Booklets, leaflets, monographs, and audiocassettes cover juvenile delinquency, drug and alcohol abuse, alienation, sex, mental health on campuses, and other topics. Payment not required with order.
INQUIRY ADDRESS. Publications Division, Hogg Foundation for Mental Health, Box 7998, University Station, University of Texas, Austin, Tex. 78712.

A134. HOSPITAL FINANCIAL MANAGEMENT ASSOCIATION, 666 N. Lake Shore Dr., Chicago, Ill. 60611. *Tel:* (312) 787-3876. R. M. Shelton, Exec. Dir.

PURPOSE. To upgrade the profession of health-care financial management. *Specialization:* financial management and accounting systems.
MEMBERSHIP. *Requirements:* must be involved in hospitals, accounting, consulting, etc. *Dues:* $52/yr.
SPECIAL INFORMATION SERVICES. Lending and reference libraries.

PUBLICATIONS. Sixteen-page publications catalog; textbooks, practice sets, manuals, compilations, career information, abstracts, American Hospital Association publications, reprints, and audiocassettes. Payment required with order under $5.

A135. HUMAN FACTORS SOCIETY, Box 1369, Santa Monica, Calif. 90406. *Tel:* (213) 394-1811. Marian G. Knowles, Exec. Asst.

PURPOSE. The exchange of information among human factors specialists. *Specialization:* human factors.
MEMBERSHIP. *Requirements:* five years experience in human factors. *Dues:* $27/yr.
PUBLICATIONS. Proceedings of meetings; *Human Factors* (bimonthly), journal; newsletter (monthly); annual directory; and indices. Films, three from Philips Electronics, and "Television Eye Marker." Payment not required with order.

A136. THE HUXLEY INSTITUTE FOR BIOSOCIAL RESEARCH—AMERICAN SCHIZOPHRENIA ASSOCIATION, 1114 First Ave., New York, N.Y. 10021. *Tel:* (212) 759-9554. Mary Ellen Roddy, Exec. Dir.

PURPOSE. A nonprofit association providing information on orthomolecular treatment for schizophrenia and related disorders. *Specialization:* orthomolecular (dietary) psychiatry.
MEMBERSHIP. *Dues:* contributing members $75; participating members $40. *Benefits:* former receive newsletter; latter, newsletter and journal.
SPECIAL INFORMATION SERVICES. Referrals to patients who are searching for an orthomolecular physician. *Special collections:* nutrition and mental illness, hyperactivity, children's learning disabilities, alcoholism, and drug abuse.
PUBLICATIONS. *Journal of Orthomolecular Psychiatry* (quarterly); newsletter (quarterly). Bibliography lists dozens of books and pamphlets repudiating Freud, advocating vitamin-filled diets. Pamphlet "Megavitamins—New Hope for the Mentally Ill." Reprints on vitamins B_3 and C treatment for mental illness. Payment required with order.

A137. ILLINOIS STATE MEDICAL SOCIETY, 55 E. Monroe, Chicago, Ill. 60603. *Tel:* (312) 782-1645. Roger N. White, Exec. Admin.

PURPOSE. A trade association of physicians pursuing education and improvement of practice, protection of health, and the well-being of the public.
PUBLICATIONS. *Illinois Medical Journal* (monthly), $8/yr. in U.S. Payment required with order.

A138. INDUSTRIAL HEALTH FOUNDATION, 5231 Centre Ave., Pittsburgh, Pa. 15232. *Tel:* (412) 687-2100. D. C. Braun, M.D., Pres.

PURPOSE. An organization of industrial concerns advancing healthful working conditions in industry. (Services restricted to member companies and nonmembers under contract.) *Specialization:* industrial medicine and toxicology.
MEMBERSHIP. *Requirements:* industrial organizations. *Dues:* $200-$2,000/yr. (scaled to size of company).

SPECIAL INFORMATION SERVICES. Literature searches (by contract to nonmembers). *Special collections: Abstracts of Occupational Health*, toxicology literature 1937–date.
PUBLICATIONS. Current reviews of occupational health programs; *Industrial Hygiene Digest* (monthly). Pamphlets; *Memos to Members*, newsletter; technical bulletins. Ten-page list of other publications in chemical engineering, toxicology, and industrial medicine. Payment required with nonmember order.

A139. INSTITUTE FOR THE STUDY OF DRUG MISUSE, 111 Fifth Ave., New York, N.Y. 10003. *Tel:* (212) 777-1000. Stanley Einstein, Exec. Dir.

PURPOSE. Concerned with education about the misuse of drugs and alcohol. *Specialization:* education on drug misuse.
MEMBERSHIP. Individuals, corporations, and organizations. *Dues:* students $7.50/yr.
SPECIAL INFORMATION SERVICES. Aid in setting up programs dealing with education about alcoholism or drug abuse; aid to sponsoring members in setting up drug/alcohol misuse department in their companies. *Special collections:* library on alcohol, drug misuse, and tobacco of over 1,000 volumes.
PUBLICATIONS. Annual monograph series *The Non-Medical Use of Drugs*; *International Journal of the Addictions* (six issues per year); *Drug Forum* (four issues per year); *American Journal of Drug and Alcohol Abuse* (four issues per year). Payment required with order.

A140. INTERNATIONAL COLLEGE OF APPLIED NUTRITION, Box 386, La Habra, Calif. 90631. *Tel:* (213) 697-4576. Mrs. Harold Stone, Exec. Sec.

PURPOSE. Concerned with postgraduate education in all phases of nutrition. *Specialization:* scientific nutrition.
MEMBERSHIP. *Requirements:* must be physician, dentist, veterinarian, or have doctorate in allied fields. *Dues:* $35/yr.
PUBLICATIONS. One booklet for lay persons; professional magazine, *Journal of Applied Nutrition* (two to three issues per year), cumulative indexes to journal. Bulletins on available fellowships. Payment required with order.

A141. INTERNATIONAL NONWOVENS AND DISPOSABLES ASSOCIA-TION, 10 E. 40 St., Room 2800, New York, N.Y. 10016. *Tel:* (212) 686-9170. Lee J. Moremen, Exec. Vice-Pres.

PURPOSE. To advance the use of nonwoven fabrics, thereby promoting growth of the industry.
SPECIAL INFORMATION SERVICES. Supplies sources for obtaining single- and limited-use products, such as surgical drapes and packs, diapers, underpads, and surgical apparel.
PUBLICATIONS. Industry directory (biannual). Payment required with order.

A142. LA LECHE LEAGUE INTERNATIONAL, INC., 9616 Minneapolis, Franklin Park, Ill. 60131. *Tel:* (312) 455-7730. Marian Tompson, Pres.

PURPOSE. A nonprofit volunteer agency established to encourage, educate, and support any mother who wishes to breastfeed her baby. Also offers breastfeeding

information to any interested person, lay or professional. *Specialization:* information, advice, coordination of group meetings of mothers, and promotion of breast-feeding.
MEMBERSHIP. All women and babies, members or not, welcome at group meetings. *Dues:* $8/yr. *Benefits:* subscription to *LLL News.*
SPECIAL INFORMATION SERVICES. Series of four meetings where women can discuss breastfeeding; personal help and encouragement from qualified league representatives; annual symposiums (accredited by ACOG and the AMA) for physicians.
PUBLICATIONS. Pamphlet "Why Nurse Your Baby?" free. Publications list of over 50 books and folders, prices ranging from 5¢ to $8.95. Large selection on physiological and psychological aspects of lactation and breastfeeding, as well as on the general fields of prenatal care and child care. Nutrition and professionally oriented topics. Most publications aimed at the nursing or undecided mother. Much of material available in braille or on tape. Pamphlets available at bulk rates. Payment not required with order.

A143. THE LALOR FOUNDATION, 4400 Lancaster Pike, Wilmington, Del. 19805. *Tel:* (302) 571-1262. C. Lalor Burdick, Ph.D., Dir. and Sec.

PURPOSE. To support research projects within a narrowly defined area of female mammalian reproductive physiology.
PUBLICATIONS. Annual announcement of grants awarded and summary of activities.

A144. MATERNITY CENTER ASSOCIATION, 48 E. 92 St., New York, N.Y. 10028. *Tel:* (212) 369-7300. Ruth Watson Lubic, Gen. Dir.

PURPOSE. To educate parents and professionals in the field of maternal and infant health. *Specialization:* maternal and infant health.
MEMBERSHIP. Contribution of $10 or more entitles membership.
SPECIAL INFORMATION Services. Phone consultation on childbearing and newborn care and for parent education.
PUBLICATIONS. Pamphlets for general audience on maternity care, childbearing, parenthood, parent education, nurse-midwifery, and teaching aids. Information for expectant mothers (on comfort during pregnancy and natural childbirth) and for expectant fathers. Center sponsors workshops and classes on childbirth and child-rearing, which are described in pamphlets. Bulk rates available. Payment not required with order.

A145. MEDICAL LIBRARY ASSOCIATION—HEALTH SCIENCES AUDIO-VISUAL GROUP, 919 N. Michigan Avenue, Chicago, Ill. 60611. *Tel:* (312) 266-2456. John LoSasso, Exec. Dir.

PURPOSE. To encourage and support audiovisual materials and their use in health sciences library programs. *Specialization:* audiovisual news and information.
MEMBERSHIP. *Requirement:* membership in Medical Library Association.
PUBLICATIONS. Media Notes in MLA *News,* free.

A146. THE MENDED HEARTS, INC., 721 Huntington Ave., Boston, Mass. 02115. *Tel:* (617) 232-9712. Emanuel Spielman, Pres.

PURPOSE. A nonprofit association to assist and encourage patients contemplating and/or recovering from heart surgery, to distribute information to patients, and to conduct and participate in research in benefit of them. (Services restricted to heart surgery patients, candidates and their families, and interested parties.)
MEMBERSHIP. *Requirements:* must have undergone or have spouse or other interested party who has undergone heart surgery.
SPECIAL INFORMATION SERVICES. *Languages:* English and Spanish.
PUBLICATIONS. *Heart Beat* (quarterly), newsletter; information pamphlets, details of visiting program. News from 70 chapters in the United States and South America. Materials free.
INQUIRY ADDRESS. 5 Scott St., Ridgefield Park, N.J. 07660. *Tel:* (201) 641-4714.

A147. MICHIGAN CANCER FOUNDATION, Meyer L. Prentiss Cancer Center, 110 E. Warren Ave., Detroit, Mich. 48201. *Tel:* (313) 833-0710. Michael J. Brennan, M.D., Pres.

PURPOSE. An agency supporting cancer research, detection, treatment, rehabilitation, public education, and public information. *Specialization:* cancer.
PUBLICATIONS. Pamphlets on breast self-examination, cancer of other parts of body (bladder, skin, etc.)—13 fact sheets in all; training kit, "Living with a Colostomy," for hospital nursing personnel (sound filmstrip); filmstrips on smoking for general public. Printed materials free. Payment for audiovisuals not required with order.

A148. NARCOTIC EDUCATIONAL FOUNDATION OF AMERICA, 5055 Sunset Blvd., Los Angeles, Calif. 90027. *Tel:* (213) 663-5171. Henry B. Hall, Exec. Sec.

PURPOSE. Concerned with narcotics education. *Specialization:* narcotics education.
SPECIAL INFORMATION SERVICES. Speakers' bureau. *Special collections:* books and pamphlets on drugs.
PUBLICATIONS. Four films aimed at youth and general audiences. Recorded statements and pamphlets on drug abuse. Payment not required with order.

A149. NATIONAL ASSOCIATION FOR HEARING AND SPEECH ACTION, 814 Thayer Ave., Silver Spring, Md. 20910. *Tel:* (301) 588-5242. Tom Coleman, Exec. Dir.

PURPOSE. To promote the interests of persons with hearing and speech handicaps and related disorders. *Specialization:* hearing and speech disorders.
PUBLICATIONS. *Washington Sounds* (monthly), newsletter; manuals on community planning for rehabilitation; audiometric training; *Hearing and Speech Action* (bimonthly), magazine; speech pathology handbooks; hearing aids; lipreading; stuttering; aphasia; booklets on history of organization and its goals. General reading for public information. Payment required with order.

A150. THE NATIONAL ASSOCIATION FOR MENTAL HEALTH, INC., 1800 N. Kent St., Arlington, Va. 22209. *Tel:* (703) 528-6405. Brian O'Connell, Exec. Dir.

PURPOSE. To stimulate citizen activity on behalf of the mentally ill to fight mental illness and promote mental health. *Specialization:* mental health.

MEMBERSHIP. Open to anyone through local Mental Health associations. *Dues:* vary from one association to another.
PUBLICATIONS. Books, pamphlets, films, videotapes, and periodicals aimed at lay people, media, and other nonprofessionals. Emphasis on consumer information. Payment required with order.

A151. NATIONAL ASSOCIATION FOR MUSIC THERAPY, INC., 901 Kentucky, No. 204, Box 610, Lawrence, Kans. 66044. *Tel:* (913) 842-1909.

PURPOSE. An association devoted to the progressive development of the use of music to accomplish therapy in hospital, educational, and community settings, and to the advancement of training and research in the music therapy profession. *Specialization:* music therapy.
MEMBERSHIP. Open to persons—professionals or volunteers—engaged in music therapy, students, organizations and institutions, and music clubs.
SPECIAL INFORMATION SERVICES. Provides information on education, curricular requirements, and lists of institutions employing music therapists.
PUBLICATIONS. *Journal of Music Therapy* (quarterly). Pamphlets on music therapy careers, advice for career counselors, and a film catalog. Latter lists five videotapes and twelve films, with content descriptions and suggested audience (therapists, doctors, college, etc.). Payment not required with institutional orders; required with individual orders.

A152. NATIONAL ASSOCIATION FOR PRACTICAL NURSE EDUCATION AND SERVICE, INC., 122 E. 42 St., New York, N.Y. 10017. *Tel:* (212) 682-3400. Lucille L. Ethridge, Exec. Dir.

PURPOSE. To develop sound practical/vocational nurse education and promote licensed nurses as important members of health team.
PUBLICATIONS. Pamphlets on career opportunities with directory of nursing programs, the association, and coronary care nursing. *Journal of Practical Nursing* (monthly). Education pamphlets and course outlines. Payment required with order.

A153. NATIONAL ASSOCIATION FOR RETARDED CITIZENS, 2709 Ave. E East, Arlington, Tex. 76011. *Tel:* (817) 261-4961. Philip Roos, Ph.D., Exec. Dir.

PURPOSE. To promote welfare of the nation's 6 million mentally retarded persons and to work to prevent incidence of mental retardation. *Specialization:* services for the mentally retarded.
MEMBERSHIP. Obtained through 1,700 local associations. *Dues:* assessed by local ARC.
SPECIAL INFORMATION SERVICES. Names and addresses of area agencies; resource bibliographies; library and reference research on topics in field of mental retardation.
PUBLICATIONS. Pamphlets, books on preventing retardation in infants, fact sheets and information on community programs; booklets on child development, day care, education, poverty, public health, retardation prevention, recreation, social work, rehabilitation, and other topics relating to the retarded. Periodicals available are *Action Together/Information Exchange* (monthly), newsletter, and *Mental Retardation News* (10 issues per year). The latter is a chatty, informative roundup, in

newspaper style, of activities around the country. Several special films are also available. Single copies free; bulk rates available. Payment required with order. INQUIRY ADDRESS. Box 6109, Arlington, Tex. 76011. *Tel:* (817) 261-4961.

A154. NATIONAL ASSOCIATION OF BLUE SHIELD PLANS, 211 E. Chicago Ave., Chicago, Ill. 60611. *Tel:* (312) 943-8181. Ned F. Parish, Pres.

PURPOSE. A national private health insurance system with public information system on health problems. *Specialization:* alcoholism, drug abuse, and suicide prevention. PUBLICATIONS. Pamphlets and films; booklets on drug and alcohol abuse and suicide. 16mm films covering same areas; one drug-abuse booklet and the film on drugs are geared toward the 4–7 age group. Material is intended for general public. Booklets are 11¢–13¢ per copy; films for sale at $75–$350 per print. Payment not required with order.

A155. NATIONAL ASSOCIATION OF CHAIN DRUG STORES, INC., 1911 Jefferson Davis Hwy., Arlington, Va. 22202. *Tel:* (703) 521-1144. Robert J. Bolger, Pres.

PURPOSE. An organization of owners of chain drugstores, providing information, communication, and legislative lobbying for the industry. *Specialization:* drugstores. MEMBERSHIP. *Requirements:* must own four drugstores or leased departments. *Dues:* from $350.
SPECIAL INFORMATION SERVICES. Industry studies.
PUBLICATIONS. Annual reports; biweekly newsletter; lobbying bulletin; *Labor Letter*, *Security Notes*, and *Drug Recall* bulletins; directories; handbooks; and other periodicals.

A156. NATIONAL ASSOCIATION OF HOSPITAL PURCHASING MANAGEMENT, 1340 N. Astor St., Suite 1201, Chicago, Ill. 60610. *Tel:* (312) 642-1082. Betty Hanna, Exec. Dir.

PURPOSE. An organization of professional hospital purchasing directors. *Specialization:* hospital purchasing.
MEMBERSHIP. *Requirements:* must be responsible for purchasing function of hospital or health-care institution.
SPECIAL INFORMATION SERVICES. Certification program, job placement, problem-solving panel, educational programs, university-oriented courses. *Special collection:* library of materials helpful to hospital purchasing managers for use of members on no-cost basis.
PUBLICATION. *Boilerplate,* newsletter (three or four issues per year). Payment required with order.

A157. NATIONAL ASSOCIATION OF RESIDENTS AND INTERNS (NARI), 292 Madison Ave., New York, N.Y. 10017. *Tel:* (212) 949-5960. George Arden, Exec. Dir.

PURPOSE. To assist members in sound economic planning through special programs and expert advice. *Specialization:* financial management. *Benefits:* free newsletter.

MEMBERSHIP. *Requirements:* M.D., D.D.S., D.M.D., or D.O. degree, interns, residents, fellows, and students. *Dues:* $12.50/yr.
PUBLICATIONS. *Stethoscope*, an irregular newsletter discussing financial management.

A158. NATIONAL BRAILLE ASSOCIATION, INC., 85 Godwin Ave., Midland Park, N.J. 07432. *Tel:* (201) 447-1484. Mrs. Irwin F. Richmond, Pres.

PURPOSE. An organization for the advancement of volunteer service to the blind and visually impaired. *Specialization:* aid to transcribers of books, etc. into braille, tape recordings, and large type.
MEMBERSHIP. *Dues:* minimum $8/yr.
PUBLICATIONS. Maintains braille book bank, largest source of college-level braille materials in the United States. Produces copies from about 1,200 masters on file and will transcribe textbooks not yet available in braille. Also on file are music scores. Separate catalogs, sent on request, list titles of books and music; printed in ink and braille editions. NBA members receive bulletin (ink, braille, and taped editions), proceedings of conferences, manuals, and instructional materials on transcribing. Nonmembers may order copies of proceedings after publication following each biennial conference. Manuals include one on tape recording, one on large-type transcribing, and dual print or braille editions of guidelines for administration of production of reading materials for visually handicapped. All available to nonmembers. Payment required with order, except by agencies and school systems.

A159. NATIONAL COUNCIL ON AGING, INC., 1828 L St. N.W., Washington, D.C. 20036.*

PURPOSE. "A nonprofit membership organization serving as a central, national resource for planning, information and materials on aging." *Specialization:* aging.
SPECIAL INFORMATION SERVICES. The NCA library is open to the public 9:30–4:30 weekdays.
PUBLICATIONS. *Current Literature on Aging* (quarterly) is an index to periodical articles on the subject; free to members; nonmembers $3/yr.

A160. NATIONAL EASTER SEAL SOCIETY FOR CRIPPLED CHILDREN AND ADULTS, 2023 W. Ogden Ave., Chicago, Ill. 60612. *Tel:* (312) 243-8400. Jayne Shover, Exec. Dir.

PURPOSE A voluntary health agency with a nationwide program of treatment, research, and education. Local societies administer rehabilitation and treatment centers, sheltered workshops, camps, and mobile and home therapy units. *Specialization:* rehabilitation, therapy, and learning disabilities.
SPECIAL INFORMATION SERVICES. Information packets assembled on request. Easter Seal Library is clearinghouse and alerts service for general public and medical professionals.
PUBLICATIONS. *Rehabilitation Literature* (monthly), professional journal on parent education, careers in rehabilitation, and learning disabilities. *Easter Seal Communicator* (ten issues per year) and annual report, both free. Thirty-six-page catalog of booklets on barrier-free design, therapy, recreation, and safety; also posters. Bulk rates available. Payment required with order under $2.

A161. NATIONAL ENVIRONMENTAL HEALTH ASSOCIATION, 1600 Pennsylvania, Denver, Colo. 80203. *Tel:* (303) 832-1550.

PURPOSE. A professional organization of workers and students involved in environmental health. *Specialization:* control of environmental hazards.
MEMBERSHIP. *Requirements:* must be employed in or studying the field of environmental health or related activities. Individual and institutional memberships.
PUBLICATIONS. *Journal of Environmental Health.* History of organization runs to 155 pages. Information on exam for registration of sanitarians/environmentalists and on environmental health curriculum. Payment not required with order.

A162. NATIONAL FEDERATION OF LICENSED PRACTICAL NURSES, 250 W. 57 St., New York, N.Y. 10019. *Tel:* (212) 246-6629. Mrs. Muriel R. Smith, Exec. Dir.

PURPOSE. A professional organization for licensed practical nurses (licensed vocational nurses) and practical nursing students, fostering high standards in education, service, and practice, and encouraging continuing education. *Specialization:* practical nursing.
MEMBERSHIP. *Requirements:* licensed practical and vocational nurses and students. *Benefits:* discounts on publications.
PUBLICATIONS. *Nursing Care* (monthly), a magainze that includes NFLPN newsletter. Pamphlets on organization, continuing education, employment opportunities, legislative lobbying, and private duty practice. Payment preferred with order.

A163. NATIONAL FOUNDATION FOR ILEITIS AND COLITIS, INC., 295 Madison Ave., New York, N.Y. 10017. *Tel:* (212) 685-3440. Irwin W. Rosenthal, Pres.

PURPOSE. An association of lay and professional people dedicated to supporting research, educating the public, and sponsoring seminars for doctors and patients on the subject of ileitis and colitis. *Specialization:* ileitis and colitis.
MEMBERSHIP. All interested people. *Dues:* $15, $25, $50, $100/yr.
PUBLICATIONS. Free pamphlets on intestinal diseases of ileitis-colitis group, information on membership, and reprints of articles in news media about the foundation and the diseases.

A164. NATIONAL FOUNDATION FOR JEWISH GENETIC DISEASES, 608 Fifth Ave., New York, N.Y. 10020. *Tel:* (212) 247-7130. George Crohn, Pres.

PURPOSE. To eradicate six known genetic diseases that affect children of predominantly Jewish heritage. Supports research and conducts public information programs. *Specialization:* Jewish genetic diseases.
SPECIAL INFORMATION SERVICES. Speaker's bureau, color slide presentation.
PUBLICATIONS. Newly established, the foundation is in the process of assembling published papers from a medical advisory board. Current information includes brochure describing the six diseases: dysautonomia, Tay-Sachs, Niemann-Pick, Blooms's syndrome, dystonia, and Gaucher's disease. Mimeographed papers on the diseases and reprints from journals. Most information free.

A165. NATIONAL FOUNDATION FOR SUDDEN INFANT DEATH, INC., 1501 Broadway, New York, N.Y. 10036. *Tel:* (212) 563-4630. Abraham B. Bergman, M.D., Pres.

PURPOSE. A non-profit volunteer health organization. *Specialization:* sudden infant death.
SPECIAL INFORMATION SERVICES. Counseling and information to parents who have lost children to sudden infant death syndrome.
PUBLICATIONS. Pamphlets and films. Payment required with order.

A166. THE NATIONAL FOUNDATION—THE MARCH OF DIMES, 1275 Mamaroneck Ave., White Plains, N.Y. 10605.

PURPOSE. To support research and dissemination of information on birth defects, their prevention, and therapy. *Specialization:* birth defects.
SPECIAL INFORMATION SERVICES. *Languages:* English and Spanish.
PUBLICATIONS. Wide range of booklets and pamphlets explaining to general public role of March of Dimes and facts about birth defects. Emphasis on perinatal care, genetic diseases, and nutrition. Three-dimensional exhibits on perinatal care. Films for loan and sound filmstrips for purchase on effects of birth defects and ways to prevent and deal with them. Single copies of publications free; bulk rates available. Payment not required with order.

A167. NATIONAL GENETICS FOUNDATION, 250 W. 57 St., New York, N.Y. 11050. *Tel:* (212) 265-3166. Ruth Berini, Exec. Dir.

PURPOSE. An agency for the referral of patients with genetic disease to network centers where they can receive diagnosis and genetic counseling. *Specialization:* genetic diseases.
SPECIAL INFORMATION SERVICES. Physicians are offered referrals and information for their patients.
PUBLICATIONS. Free pamphlets describing the network of genetic counseling centers and problems that could be expected with pregnancies after age 35. Also reprints of articles on expanding science of treating genetic defects.

A168. THE NATIONAL HEMOPHILIA FOUNDATION, 25 W. 39 St., New York, N.Y. 10018. *Tel:* (212) 869-9740. George J. Theobald, Jr., Exec. Dir.

PURPOSE. A voluntary nonprofit organization, charter member of World Federation of Hemophilia, and member of National Health Council. Supports research and distributes information and educational materials. *Specialization:* hemophilia.
MEMBERSHIP. *Requirements:* varies by chapter.
PUBLICATIONS. "Hemofax" (monthly), newsletter; materials for door-to-door collectors; publicity aids; TV spots; slides; radio tapes; educational literature with bulk rates; and fundraising aids. Payment not required with order.

A169. NATIONAL LUPUS ERYTHEMATOSUS FOUNDATION, INC., 5430 Van Nuys Blvd., No. 206, Van Nuys, Calif. 91401. *Tel:* (213) 885-8787. Tom Bane, Chmn. of the Board.

PURPOSE. A nonprofit volunteer organization that distributes literature, compiles information from patients, funds research, and aids in establishing chapters dealing with lupus erythematosus. *Specialization:* lupus erythematosus.
MEMBERSHIP. Open to all interested persons.
PUBLICATIONS. Pamphlets and handouts on symptoms and characteristics of lupus erythematosus, a chronic disease affecting mainly young women. Information on research programs, centering around Los Angeles-University of Southern California Medical Center. Most material free.

A170. NATIONAL MULTIPLE SCLEROSIS SOCIETY, 257 Park Ave. S., New York, N.Y. 10010. *Tel:* (212) 674-4100. Sylvia Lawry, Exec. Dir.

PURPOSE. A voluntary health agency engaged in support of research to find cause, prevention, and cure of multiple sclerosis. Programs include research, community and patient services, professional education, and public information.
MEMBERSHIP. Contributory memberships.
PUBLICATIONS. Materials for professionals include works reprinted from journals on all aspects of diagnosis and treatment. Other materials for general public include annual report, *MS Messenger* (quarterly), and *MS Briefs* (for chapters). For patients and their families are booklets on learning to live with multiple sclerosis and information on research. Two medical films available—one on research for general audiences and one on diagnosis for medical professionals and students. Educational films include segment shown on "Marcus Welby, M.D." TV series; others on how multiple sclerosis affects victims. Contact local chapter for ordering information.

A171. NATIONAL PUBLIC RELATIONS COUNCIL OF HEALTH AND WELFARE SERVICES, INC., 815 Second Ave., New York, N.Y. 10017. *Tel:* (212) 687-1223. Don Bates, Exec. Dir.

PURPOSE. To improve communications and public relations in behalf of public and private programs serving health, social welfare, and human services needs. (Services restricted to organizational and sustaining members.) *Specialization:* public relations in nonprofit organizations, fundraising, and institute presentations.
MEMBERSHIP. Open to all interested people. Three categories of membership with corresponding levels of dues. *Benefits:* twice monthly newsletter, loan library, discounts, and consultation and evaluation services.
SPECIAL INFORMATION SERVICES. Loan library of print materials and how-to instructions in communications and public relations; consultation and evaluation of print materials and public relations-communications plans. *Special collections:* public relations-communications in health organizations.
PUBLICATIONS. Pamphlets, audiotapes, and periodicals. Payment required with order.

A172. NATIONAL REHABILITATION ASSOCIATION, 1522 K St. N.W., Washington, D.C. 20005. Lowell E. Green, Pres.

PURPOSE. To rehabilitate all handicapped persons. *Specialization:* rehabilitation of the handicapped.

MEMBERSHIP. Professional workers in rehabilitation and others interested in problems of the handicapped.
PUBLICATIONS. *Journal of Rehabilitation*, *NRA Newsletter*, and *Legislative Newsletter*.

A173. NATIONAL SAFETY COUNCIL, 4255 N. Michigan Ave., Chicago, Ill. 60611. *Tel:* (312) 527-4800. Vincent L. Tofany, Pres.

PURPOSE. Concerned with safety and accident prevention. *Specialization:* accident prevention.
PUBLICATIONS. Accident Prevention Manual for Industrial Operations; illustrated 72-page catalog and poster directory. Films, manuals, and technical publications; slides; leaflets; awards; newsletters; and stickers. Payment required with order under $5.

A174. NATIONAL SOCIETY FOR THE PREVENTION OF BLINDNESS, INC., 79 Madison Ave., New York, N.Y. 10016. *Tel:* (212) 684-3505. Mrs. Boyce, Exec. Dir.

PURPOSE. To determine causes of and eliminate preventable blindness. *Specialization:* eye safety and blindness.
SPECIAL INFORMATION SERVICES. *Special collections:* current publications on vision and vision problems. Many technical volumes and archives for handling correspondence.
PUBLICATIONS. Publications and 12-page film catalog describe materials on diseases and other eye problems of children and adults; eye safety; references; publications of professional interest; safety incentive program; 18 films for purchase or rent on glaucoma, cataracts, and eye safety. Many single copies free. Payment not required with order.
INQUIRY ADDRESS. Publications Department, National Association for the Prevention of Blindness, Inc., 79 Madison Ave., New York, N.Y. 10016. *Tel:* (212) 684-3505, ext. 25/26.

A175. NORTH CAROLINA SAFETY CONFERENCE, 4000 Old Wake Forest Rd., Raleigh, N.C. 27611. *Tel:* (919) 829-4820. Robert K. Adams II, Dir. of Safety.

PURPOSE. A branch of the North Carolina Industrial Commission dealing with accident prevention services and a sponsor of regional safety councils. (Services restricted to North Carolina industry.) *Specialization:* safety and accident education and prevention.
PUBLICATIONS. *Safety Bulletins* (quarterly). Safety film library. All services free.

A176. THE NUTRITION FOUNDATION, INC., 489 Fifth Ave., New York, N.Y. 10017. *Tel:* (212) 687-4830. Dr. William J. Darby, Pres.

PURPOSE. Concerned with nutrition education from general to professional levels and support of research in nutrition and related fields. *Specialization:* nutrition.
PUBLICATIONS. Pamphlets on proper eating; medical and scientific books; mono-

graphs; results of symposia; and indexes and bibliographies. Monthly journal. Payment not required with order.

INQUIRY ADDRESS. 888 17 St. N.W., Washington, D.C. 20006. *Tel:* (202) 872-0778.

A177. OPTICAL SOCIETY OF AMERICA, 2000 L St. N.W., Washington, D.C. 20036. *Tel:* (202) 293-1420. Jarus W. Quinn, Exec. Dir.

PURPOSE. To increase and diffuse knowledge of optics. *Specialization:* optics.
MEMBERSHIP. *Requirements:* appropriate training or experience in optics. *Dues:* $30/yr. *Benefits:* publications for members and participation in technical meetings.
PUBLICATIONS. *Journal of the Optical Society of America* (paper and microfiche editions); *Optics News* (quarterly); *Applied Optics*; translations of Soviet journals *Optika i spektroskopiya* and *Optikomechanicheskaya promyshlennost*; indices and supplements to journals. Books and digests of meetings. Payment not required with order.

A178. THE ORTON SOCIETY, INC., 8415 Bellona Lane, Suite 817, Towson, Md. 21204. *Tel:* (301) 296-0232. N. Dale Bryant, Ph.D., Pres.

PURPOSE. To disseminate educational information concerning specific language disabilities. *Specialization:* dyslexia.
MEMBERSHIP. Open to all interested in the field of specific language disabilities. *Dues:* individual $15/yr.; full-time student $5/yr.
PUBLICATIONS. Books, monographs, bibliographies, and over 60 reprints of papers, covering speech problems, word blindness, dyslexia, underachievement, remedial training, and other aspects of reading and speech disability. *Bulletin of the Orton Society* (annual). Payment required with order.

A179. PARENTERAL DRUG ASSOCIATION, INC., 1206 Western Savings Bank Building, Broad and Chestnut St., Philadelphia, Pa. 19107. *Tel:* (215) 735-9752. H. E. Boyden, Admin. Sec.

PURPOSE. A technical and professional organization, including manufacturers of sterile pharmaceuticals, college faculty, biochemists, microbiologists, and others. *Specialization:* parenteral drugs.
MEMBERSHIP. *Dues:* individual $35/yr.; corporate $200/yr.
PUBLICATIONS. Annotated bibliographies on parenteral dosage forms. Slide/sound program, "Sterile Products and You," aimed at employees of hospitals and sterile-environment industries. Bimonthly bulletin for members. Payment required with order.

A180. PARKINSON'S DISEASE FOUNDATION, INC., 640 W. 168 St., New York, N.Y. 10032. *Tel:* (212) WA 3-4700. H. Houston Merritt, M.D., Pres.

PURPOSE. To support research in Parkinson's disease and to distribute pertinent literature. Also serves as an information source for patients and doctors. *Specialization:* Parkinson's disease.
SPECIAL INFORMATION SERVICES. Progress on research, referrals to clinics and neurologists, and literature for patients and families.
PUBLICATIONS. Pamphlets on Parkinson's disease. Information on coping with

disease; exercise booklet for victims, and reprint on L-dopa treatment; *The Parkinson Patient at Home.* Payment not required with order.
INQUIRY ADDRESS. 640 W. 168 St., New York, N.Y. 10032. *Tel:* (212) WA 3-7800.

A181. PHARMACEUTICALS MANUFACTURERS ASSOCIATION, 1155 15 St. N.W., Washington, D.C. 20005. *Tel:* (202) 296-2440. C. Joseph Stetler, Pres.

PURPOSE. An organization of drug makers to promote high standards in products, encourage research and disseminate information to and on behalf of drug makers. (Services restricted to member firms.) *Specialization:* health education and prescription medicines.
MEMBERSHIP. *Requirements:* firms. *Dues:* based on sales volume.
SPECIAL INFORMATION SERVICES. Speaker's bureau, including representatives of leading drug manufacturers.
PUBLICATIONS. Consumer information in pamphlet form, purchased in lots of 100; drug abuse information—symptoms, how to educate about abuse; general information on happenings in the industry, legislatures; also newsletter, bulletin, commentaries, surveys of industry, annual report, and other topics. Payment not required with order.

A182. THE PHYSICIANS FORUM, INC., 510 Madison Ave., New York, N.Y. 10022. *Tel:* (212) 688-3290. Patricia Lievow, Exec. Sec.

PURPOSE. A professional organization of physicians working for a national health service with a single class of medical care for all, financed by progressive income tax surcharge for health. *Specialization:* health-care reform.
MEMBERSHIP. To physicians, medical students, and nonphysicians. *Dues:* $10–$100/yr.
PUBLICATIONS. Informational pamphlets on inadequacy of nation's health-care delivery system and need for drastic change. Information on drug prices, physician training, hospital costs, as well as other topics. Payment required with large order.

A183. PIERRE FAUCHARD ACADEMY, 4015 W. 65 St., Minneapolis, Minn. 55435. *Tel:* (612) 927-7965.

PURPOSE. A dental organization promoting education through literature. (Services restricted to dentists and oral physicians.) *Specialization:* dentistry.
MEMBERSHIP. *Requirements:* must be ADA member and pay dues.
PUBLICATIONS. *Dental World* (quarterly), $4/yr. Payment required with order.

A184. PLANNED PARENTHOOD FEDERATION OF AMERICA, 810 Seventh Ave., New York, N.Y. 10019. *Tel:* (212) 541-7800. Jack Hood Vaughn, Pres.

PURPOSE. To assist individuals to have control over their own fertility and to help bring about orderly transition to zero population growth. *Specialization:* family planning, health education, professional information, and fund-raising.
SPECIAL INFORMATION SERVICES. *Languages:* English and Spanish.
PUBLICATIONS. Numerous, including magazine *Family Planning Perspectives* (bimonthly); *Washington Memo* (at least 20 issues per year), news from federal government; *Family Planning/Population Reporter* (bimonthly). Bibliographic

brochure with English and Spanish listings; monthly bibliography, *Current Literature in Family Planning*, lists new books and articles on contraceptive research, sexuality, and child care and health. Film catalog with selections on abortion, birth control methods, population problems, counseling, sex education, sterilization, dating, and marriage. Also slides, records, and audiotapes. Payment not required with order.

INQUIRY ADDRESS. Publications Section, Planned Parenthood Federation of America, 810 Seventh Ave., New York, N.Y. 10019. *Tel:* (212) 541-7800.

A185. POPULATION ASSOCIATION OF AMERICA, Box 14182, Benjamin Franklin Station, Washington, D.C. 20044.

PURPOSE. A scientific and professional society "to promote the improvement, advancement, and progress of the human race by means of research with respect to problems connected with human population, in both its quantitative and qualitative aspects, and the dissemination and publication of the results of this research. . . ." *Specialization:* demography; family planning; marriage, divorce, and the family; methods of research and analysis; and statistics, censuses, and surveys.

MEMBERSHIP. Everyone interested in the field of population. Special memberships for husband-and-wife teams, students, and organizations. *Benefits:* members receive publications free.

PUBLICATIONS. *Demography* (quarterly); *Population Index* (quarterly) published by Office of Population Research, Princeton University; and *PAA Affairs* (quarterly), newsletter.

A186. POPULATION REFERENCE BUREAU, INC., 1755 Massachusetts Ave. N.W., Washington, D.C. 20036. *Tel:* (202) 232-2288. Robert M. Avedon, Pres.

PURPOSE. To gather, interpret, and publish information on population dynamics and their implications for social and economic development, the environment, and resources. *Specialization:* population, demography, and population education.

MEMBERSHIP. Institutions, individuals, libraries, teachers, and students. *Dues:* $2–$50.

SPECIAL INFORMATION SERVICES. Collection of U.S. censuses going back to colonial times, reference and information service in area of population. *Special collections:* journals in population and family planning, public health, family counseling, and environment.

PUBLICATIONS. *Interchange* newsletter lists latest publications from bureau, workshops, and other events. Bureau produces steady output of bulletins and pamphlets on world trends in birth rates, death rates, nutrition, aging, government population policies, abortion, birth control, and demography. *Population Bulletin* (bimonthly), *World Population Data Sheet* (annual). Bulk rates available on publications. *PRB Report* gives chronology of major events in world population control during 1973–1974. Attractive wall charts include country-by-country rundown on vital population statistics. Payment required with order.

A187. PROFESSIONAL REHABILITATION WORKERS WITH THE ADULT DEAF, 814 Thayer Ave., Silver Spring, Md. 20910. *Tel:* (301) 589-0880. Chas. R. Hill, Exec. Sec.

PURPOSE. To promote development and expansion of professional rehabilitation services for the adult deaf. *Specialization:* rehabilitation of deaf adults.
MEMBERSHIP. Must be professional in field of providing services on behalf of deaf adults—counselor, social worker, audiologist, speech therapist, etc. *Dues:* $25/yr. *Benefits:* subscription to journal and other publications.
PUBLICATIONS. *Journal of Rehabilitation of the Deaf* (quarterly); periodic newsletter; pamphlets. Payment not required with order.

A188. PUBLIC AFFAIRS COMMITTEE, 381 Park Ave. S., New York, N.Y. 10016. *Tel:* (212) 683-4331. Maxwell S. Stewart, Sec.

PURPOSE. An organization distributing pamphlets on social and health problems. *Specialization:* health and social problems.
SPECIAL INFORMATION SERVICES. *Languages:* English and Spanish.
PUBLICATIONS. Pamphlets on population, marijuana, retardation, homosexuality, noise, and drug abuse. Health materials, aimed at general audiences, deal with sex education, accident prevention, first aid, suicide, and chronic illnesses. Films on importance of immunization of children and prenatal care. Payment required with order under $5.

A189. RECOVERY, INCORPORATED—THE ASSOCIATION OF NERVOUS AND FORMER MENTAL PATIENTS, 116 S. Michigan Ave., Chicago, Ill. 60614. *Tel:* (312) 263-2292. Robert L. Farwell, Exec. Dir.

PURPOSE. To offer at weekly group meetings demonstrations of the recovery method of self-help after-care in order to help prevent relapses in former mental patients and chronic symptoms in nervous patients. *Specialization:* help "for those who want to help themselves" in preventing relapses or chronicity of nervous disorders and mental illnesses.
MEMBERSHIP. Loose structure of organization puts most emphasis on self-help. Weekly meetings held at some 1,000 locations in the United States, Canada, and Puerto Rico. Meetings open to all. *Dues:* none, contributions from participants are accepted.
PUBLICATIONS. Books by Dr. Abraham Low, founder, including *Mental Health Through Will Training*—required reading for recovery members participating at meetings. Informational pamphlets; national directory of meeting places; recorded lectures by Low (records of cassettes) also available. *The Recovery Reporter* sent to members every two months. Information on membership free; payment for other literature required with order.

A190. REHABILITATION INTERNATIONAL, USA, 20 W. 40 St., New York, N.Y. 10018. *Tel:* (212) 869-9907. Ellis Reida, Exec. Dir.

PURPOSE. To gather information from around world for use of rehabilitation community in the United States. Engages in publishing and runs film library. (Services restricted to U.S. rehabilitation community.) *Specialization:* rehabilitation.
MEMBERSHIP. *Dues:* $15/yr. *Benefits:* members receive two rehabilitation reviews.
SPECIAL INFORMATION SERVICES. Information on barrier-free design, sheltered

workshops, architectural barriers. *Languages:* films in English, Japanese, Hebrew, and German.

PUBLICATIONS. *Rehabilitation/WORLD* (quarterly) and *International Rehabilitation Review*. Film catalog runs to 40 pages; lists 250 films from the United States, Canada, Britain, Japan, and other countries. Plans are afoot to add 8mm films and also videotapes to current stock of exclusively 16mm fields. Films are for rent for modest fee, about $10. Topics include deafness, employment, public health, and the aged. Publications only for dues-paying members. Payment not required with order.

A191. ST. LOUIS ASSOCIATION FOR RETARDED CHILDREN, 6372 Clayton Rd., St. Louis, Mo. 63117. *Tel:* (314) 647-5190. Richard I. Goldbaum, Exec. Dir.

PURPOSE. To serve mentally retarded citizens and their families.
SPECIAL INFORMATION SERVICES. Family education, counseling by social workers, referrals to agencies, speaker's bureau. Runs recreation programs, day and residence camps, counseling and referral services.
PUBLICATIONS. Pamphlets describe services and aims. New film, *On Being Sexual*, explores sexuality and the mentally retarded, with parents and professionals speaking on topic; accompanied by guidebook; for rent or purchase. Payment required with order.
INQUIRY ADDRESS. 1240 Dautel Lane. *Tel:* (314) 569-2211.

A192. SMART FAMILY FOUNDATION, 65 E. South Water St., Chicago, Ill. 60601.*

PURPOSE. A philanthropic organization offering films for medical groups. *Specialization:* medical films.
PRODUCTS. Films on patient education, child psychology, and other topics are offered to health institutions, training facilities, and community groups. Free.

A193. SOCIETY FOR NUTRITION EDUCATION, 2140 Shattuck Ave., Suite 1110, Berkeley, Calif. 94704. *Tel:* (415) 548-1363. Helen D. Ullrich, Exec. Dir.

PURPOSE. A professional society dedicated to promoting good nutrition by making nutrition education more effective. Engages in education, communication, and research. (Services restricted to members.) *Specialization:* nutrition education.
MEMBERSHIP. *Requirements:* voting members must have B.S. degree and training or experience in nutrition education. Nonvoting memberships available for students and others.
SPECIAL INFORMATION SERVICES. Preparation of bibliographies and review of educational projects; consultants in the field.
PUBLICATIONS. Pamphlets and periodicals, including *Journal of Nutrition Education*. Payment required with order.
INQUIRY ADDRESS. Sue Ellen Rowe, National Nutrition Education Clearing House, 2140 Shattuck Ave., Suite 1110, Berkeley, Calif. 94704. *Tel:* (415) 548-1363.

A194. SOCIETY FOR RESEARCH IN CHILD DEVELOPMENT, INC., 5801 S. Ellis Ave., Chicago, Ill. 60637. *Tel:* (312) 753-3370. Dorothy H. Eichorn, Exec. Off.

PURPOSE. An association for advancing research, fostering interdisciplinary consideration of substantive and methodological problems, and encouraging study of implications of research findings for instruction in child development. *Specialization:* child development.
MEMBERSHIP. *Requirements:* membership open to those actively engaged in research in child development or in basic sciences related to it and who teach graduate or undergraduate courses in child development. *Dues:* $24/yr.; graduate students $18/yr.
PUBLICATIONS. *Child Development* (quarterly), *Child Development Abstracts and Bibliography* (triannual), and *Monographs of the Society for Research in Child Development.* Also books and audiotapes. Payment required with order.

A195. SOCIETY OF GENERAL PHYSIOLOGISTS, Box 257, Woods Hole, Mass. 02543. Joe Hoffman, Pres.

PURPOSE. To promote research in general physiology. *Specialization:* general physiology.
MEMBERSHIP. *Requirements:* must be active in research. *Dues:* $8/yr.
PUBLICATIONS. Books (through Raven Press), newsletter for members, *Journal of General Physiology* (through Rockefeller Press).

A196. SOCIETY OF TOXICOLOGY, Esso Research and Engineering Co., Box 45, Linden, N.J. 07036. *Tel:* (201) 474-2422. Robert A. Scala, Sec.

PURPOSE. A professional society promoting knowledge in toxicology. (Services restricted to members and professional or government organizations.) *Specialization:* toxicology.
MEMBERSHIP. *Requirements:* open to persons with continuing professional interest in toxicology or with research or expertise in the field.
PUBLICATIONS. *Toxicology and Applied Pharmacology* (monthly), journal. Order from Academic Press, 111 Fifth Ave., New York, N.Y. 10003.

A197. SOUTHERN MEDICAL ASSOCIATION, 2601 Highland Ave., Birmingham, Ala. 35205.* *Tel:* (205) 324-4608. Andrew M. Moore, M.D., Pres.

PURPOSE. A professional organization of physicians in the southeastern United States. *Specialization:* audiotapes for medical professionals.
PUBLICATIONS. "Medical Playback" series of audiocassettes for medical professionals, recorded at SMA annual scientific meetings. Payment not required with order.

A198. SOUTHERN REGIONAL EDUCATION BOARD, 130 Sixth St. N.W., Atlanta, Ga. 30313. *Tel:* (404) 875-9211. Dr. W. L. Godwin, Pres.

PURPOSE. An association to promote regional planning for educational program development. *Specialization:* nursing, mental health, human services, optometry, and health manpower.
PUBLICATIONS. Pamphlets and periodicals. Free *Regional Spotlight* (quarterly) usually devotes one issue every year to health. Book on regional plan for expanding optometric education in the South, $4. *Nursing Research in the South* and *Workbook on the Environments for Nursing*; both free. Payment required with order.

A199. SPECIAL LIBRARIES ASSOCIATION, 235 Park Ave. S., New York, N.Y. 10003.* *Tel:* (212) 777-8136.

PURPOSE. An association for librarians in special libraries, which include, among others, medical, scientific, technical, pharmaceutical, and business libraries. *Specialization:* publications for the special library.

PUBLICATIONS. Books include directories, bibliographies, subject heading lists, and professional literature for the special librarian on planning and personnel. Periodicals and indexes include scientific meetings, special libraries, technical book review index, translations register-index, and information science abstracts. Discounts are available to institutions. Payment required with individual order.

TAKE OFF POUNDS SENSIBLY *See* A200

A200. TOPS (TAKE OFF POUNDS SENSIBLY) CLUB, INC., 4575 S. Fifth St., Milwaukee, Wisc. 53209. *Tel:* (414) 482-4620. Esther S. Manz, Pres.

PURPOSE. A nonprofit organization of weight-control clubs. *Specialization:* weight control.

MEMBERSHIP. *Dues:* $7/yr. for first two years; $5/yr. after. *Benefits:* members use diets prescribed by personal physicians.

PUBLICATIONS. *TOPS News* (monthly), magazine for members; pamphlets; bibliography of medical and scientific papers out of obesity and metabolic research program. Payment not required with order.

A201. ZERO POPULATION GROWTH, INC., 1346 Connecticut Ave. N.W., Washington, D.C. 20036. *Tel:* (202) 785-0100. Robert Dennis, Exec. Dir.

PURPOSE. To promote population stabilization, to be followed by gradual reduction in population, in the United States by voluntary means. *Specialization:* population.

MEMBERSHIP. *Dues:* students $8/yr.; general $15/yr. *Benefits:* Members receive *ZPG Reporter*.

PUBLICATIONS. *ZPG National Reporter* (ten issues per year), $5.50/yr. Pamphlets on population growth and stabilization. Payment required with order.

B

Audiovisual Producers and Distributors

ABBOTT LABORATORIES *See* F1

ACADEMIC PRESS, INC./GRUNE & STRATTON, INC. *See* G1

B1. ACI FILMS, INC., 35 W. 45 St., New York, N.Y. 10036.* *Tel:* (212) 582-1918. Stelios Roccos, Pres.

PURPOSE. Producer of multimedia instructional programs for the classroom. *Specialization:* sales of multimedia classroom materials.
PUBLICATIONS. Catalogs for 16mm films and sound filmstrips are illustrated and make good reference material. Filmstrips cover health and safety for primary and elementary grades, treat drugs and pollution and venereal disease. For higher grades, subjects include life sciences, basic biology, and growing up. Programs come with study guides; some films can be captioned. Payment not required with order.

B2. AETNA LIFE AND CASUALTY, Public Relations and Advertising Department, 151 Farmington Ave., Hartford, Conn. 06115.*

PURPOSE. An insurance company with health advisories for the general public. *Specialization:* health and safety.
PUBLICATIONS. Pamphlets outline dangers of drinking, importance of safety, and the ever-present danger of child poisoning. Film list (for free loan to organizations), some films also on 3/4" videotape, portray child poisoning, alcoholism in industry (directed toward managers and superintendents), and other topics for the general public. "Tuffy Talks About Medicine," a coloring book for toddlers and the young at heart, teaches dangers of indiscriminate pill-taking by children.

B3. AGENCY FOR INSTRUCTIONAL TELEVISION (AIT), Box A, 1111 W. 17 St., Bloomington, Ind. 47401. *Tel:* (812) 339-2203. Edwin G. Cohen, Exec. Dir.

PURPOSE. An American-Canadian organization to develop and coordinate cooperative educational programs with state and provincial agencies. Also acquires, adapts, and distributes television, audiovisual and printed materials for use as learning resources. (Services restricted to schools and school systems, educational TV stations, and other educational organizations.)
PUBLICATIONS. Lively, illustrated catalogs. *Guide Book* lists purposes and ongoing projects of AIT, along with available television courses. *Inside Out* is collection of 30, 15-minute programs in emotional health education for 8- to 10-year-olds. *Self, Incorporated* is similar project aimed at the 11-to-13 age group. Quarterly newsletter (illustrated and well produced) available free of charge to interested persons and organizations. Payment not required with order.

B4. AIMS INSTRUCTIONAL MEDIA SERVICES, INC., Box 1010, Hollywood, Calif. 90028. *Tel:* (213) 467-1171. Charles Cahill, Pres.

PURPOSE. To distribute wide variety of educational films and filmstrips to school and nonschool clients. *Specialization:* films and filmstrips on all subjects.
PUBLICATIONS. Well-illustrated 28-page filmstrip catalog on health, safety and life sciences for school-age viewers. Similar topics covered in 76-page film catalog that also lists some sound filmstrips. Good selections, well described. Payment not required with order.

B5. ALBANY MEDICAL COLLEGE, Department of Postgraduate Medicine, Albany, N.Y. 12208.*

PURPOSE. To produce audiovisual programs for institutional use in training health professionals. *Specialization:* AV programs for health professionals.
PUBLICATIONS. Audiocassettes, tapes, and slides explore allergies, diagnoses, infectious diseases, musculoskeletal system, poisoning and injury, psychiatry, pulmonary diseases, and sociomedical problems (such as drug abuse, battered children, methadone maintenance, death and dying). Payment not required with order.

ALDINE PUBLISHING COMPANY *See* G4

ALFRED ADLER INSTITUTE OF CHICAGO *See* G5

B6. ALFRED HIGGINS PRODUCTIONS, INC., 9100 Sunset Blvd., Los Angeles, Calif. 90069. *Tel:* (213) 878-0330. Alfred Higgins, Pres.

PURPOSE. To produce and distribute educational films. *Specialization:* production of educational films.
PUBLICATIONS. Catalog lists general-audience films on the importance of good nutrition, personal hygiene, and dangers of tobacco, drugs, and venereal disease. The nine films in the field of health are aimed at elementary to senior high school audiences. New films tell of physiological harm from excessive noise, and one is designed to allay children's fear of hospitals. Films are for purchase. Payment not required with order.

B7. ALTERNATE VISIONS, INC., 130 W. 86 St., New York, N.Y. 10024.*

PURPOSE. To produce videotapes on social issues. *Specialization:* videotapes. PUBLICATIONS. Tapes illustrate British method of treating heroin addiction, problems of ex-addicts, introduction to acupuncture, and resistance among mental patients to pressures in institutions for their treatment. Payment not required with order.

ALTON OCHSNER MEDICAL FOUNDATION *See* A7

AMERICAN ACADEMY OF OPHTHALMOLOGY AND OTOLARYNGOLOGY—CONTINUING EDUCATION WITH TELEVISION *See* A13

AMERICAN ACADEMY OF ORAL PATHOLOGY *See* A15

AMERICAN ACADEMY OF ORTHOPAEDIC SURGEONS *See* A16

AMERICAN ASSOCIATION FOR MATERNAL AND CHILD HEALTH, INC. *See* A20

AMERICAN ASSOCIATION FOR THE ADVANCEMENT OF SCIENCE *See* A22

AMERICAN ASSOCIATION OF BLOOD BANKS *See* A25

AMERICAN ASSOCIATION OF COLLEGES OF PHARMACY *See* A26

AMERICAN BAR ASSOCIATION *See* A33

AMERICAN CANCER SOCIETY *See* A34

AMERICAN CHEMICAL SOCIETY *See* A35

AMERICAN CHIROPRACTIC ASSOCIATION *See* A36

AMERICAN COLLEGE HEALTH ASSOCIATION *See* A37

AMERICAN COLLEGE OF CARDIOLOGY EXTENDED LEARNING *See* A38

AMERICAN COLLEGE OF RADIOLOGY *See* A40

AMERICAN COLLEGE OF SURGEONS *See* A41

AMERICAN COLLEGE OF SURGEONS FILM LIBRARY *See* A42

AMERICAN DENTAL ASSOCIATION, BUREAU OF DENTAL HEALTH ASSOCIATION *See* A46

B8. AMERICAN EDUCATIONAL FILMS, INC., 132 Lasky Dr., Beverly Hills, Calif. 90212. *Tel:* (213) 278-4996. Robert Springer, Pres.

PURPOSE. To produce and distribute films. *Specialization:* films on health and science.

PUBLICATIONS. Sixteen-page catalog. Health films are for general audiences, covering venereal disease, family planning, first aid, alcohol and other drugs, and mental illness. All films listed are also available as videocassettes. Study guide with each film/cassette.

B9. AMERICAN FILM PRODUCTIONS, INC., 1540 Broadway, New York, N.Y. 10036. *Tel:* (212) 582-1900. Robert Gross, Pres.

PURPOSE. To produce motion pictures. *Specialization:* safety films.

PUBLICATIONS. Emphasis on safety and first aid—upper airway obstruction, prevention of sports injuries, water safety, diving injuries, and drownproofing. Also sound filmstrips. Payment not required with order.

AMERICAN FOUNDATION FOR THE BLIND *See* A49

AMERICAN INSTITUTE OF THE HISTORY OF PHARMACY *See* A55

AMERICAN JOURNAL OF NURSING COMPANY *See* G8

AMERICAN LUNG ASSOCIATION *See* A57

AMERICAN MEDICAL RECORD ASSOCIATION *See* A59

AMERICAN MEDICAL STUDENT ASSOCIATION *See* A60

AMERICAN OCCUPATIONAL THERAPY ASSOCIATION *See* A64

AMERICAN OPTOMETRIC ASSOCIATION *See* A65

AMERICAN OSTEOPATHIC ASSOCIATION *See* A67

AMERICAN PHARMACEUTICAL ASSOCIATION *See* A68

AMERICAN PHYSIOLOGICAL SOCIETY *See* A70

AMERICAN PODIATRY ASSOCIATION *See* A71

AMERICAN PROTESTANT HOSPITAL ASSOCIATION *See* A73

AMERICAN SOCIETY FOR HOSPITAL PERSONNEL ADMINISTRATION *See* A83

AMERICAN SOCIETY OF ABDOMINAL SURGEONS *See* A87

AMERICAN SOCIETY OF CLINICAL PATHOLOGISTS *See* A89

AMERICAN SOCIETY OF HEMATOLOGY *See* A90

AMERICAN THORACIC SOCIETY *See* A96

AMERICAN VETERINARY MEDICAL ASSOCIATION *See* A97

B10. AMERICAN VIDEO NETWORK, 660 S. Bonnie Brae, Los Angeles, Calif. 90057. *Tel:* (213) 483-6220. Dr. Norman Traverse, Pres.

PURPOSE. To distribute videotape programs. (Services restricted to hospitals, colleges, and businesses.) *Specialization:* videotapes on health care, education, and business.
PUBLICATIONS. Color videotape cassettes on nurses' training, including about 20 on patient care, emergencies, cleaning, and diet. Also extensive videocassette program in continuing medical education, with series on internal medicine, critical care, family practice, ophthalmology, surgery, pathology, and other fields. Videotape or film on emergency childbirth, as well as crisis intervention, quitting tobacco, and educating the patient. Payment not required with order.

B11. ARIZONA STATE UNIVERSITY, Media Research and Development, Tempe, Ariz. 85281.*

PURPOSE. A media production center. *Specialization:* audiovisual production.
PUBLICATIONS. Multimedia programs demonstrate how to produce effective audiovisual presentations—planning, graphics, photography, copying, sound, and presentation. Series designed for those in media and in other professions. Complete series $90. Payment not required with order.

ARKANSAS DEPARTMENT OF HEALTH *See* D3

ARMED FORCES INSTITUTE OF PATHOLOGY *See* D4

B12. ARNOLD EAGLE PRODUCTIONS, 41 W. 47 St., New York, N.Y. 10036. *Tel:* (212) JU 2-4248. Arnold Eagle, Owner.

PURPOSE. To produce films. *Specialization:* educational films.
PUBLICATIONS. *Diary of Connie McGregor,* chronicle of the experiences of a nursing student. Payment not required with order.

ARTHRITIS FOUNDATION *See* A98

B13. ASPECT II EDUCATIONAL FILMS, 21 Charles St., Westport, Conn. 06880.* *Tel:* (203) 227-5544.

PURPOSE. To produce educational films for children. *Specialization:* children's films.
PUBLICATIONS. Films include *The People Shop,* 16mm sound-color, which "presents the community hospital as a real and integral part of the community and its life." Purchase $220; rental $22. Payment not required with order.

ASSOCIATION FOR THE ADVANCEMENT OF HEALTH EDUCATION *See* A100

B14. ASSOCIATION INSTRUCTIONAL MATERIALS, 866 Third Avenue, New York, N.Y. 10022.* *Tel:* (212) 935-4210. Robert D. Mitchell, Pres.

PURPOSE. The sale and rental of educational films on education, health, and welfare. *Specialization:* educational films.
PUBLICATIONS. One-hundred-and-twenty-page catalog. Good psychology selection, touching on mental retardation and behavior, including "Dynamics of Leadership" series for effective group action and series on "Personality." Warnings on drug abuse; advisories on good grooming and charm; obesity, health-care delivery to the inner city; alarmist views of alternative lifestyles (*From Runaway to Hippie*); and smoking and alcohol. For elementary and high school levels. Payment not required with order.

ASSOCIATION FOR THE STUDY OF ABORTION *See* A101

ASTRA PHARMACEUTICAL PRODUCTS *See* F2

ATHLETIC INSTITUTE *See* A106

B15. AUDIO AND VISUAL METHODS COMPANY, Box 8593, Rochester, N.Y. 14619.* *Tel:* (716) 328-8354.

PURPOSE. To provide visual teaching aids for medical professionals and paraprofessionals. *Specialization:* audiovisual classroom aids.
PUBLICATIONS. Filmstrips; super-8 loops produced by Camera Talk, Ltd. of London—intended as supplements to classroom texts. Payment not required with order.

B16. AUDIO-DIGEST FOUNDATION, 1930 Wilshire Blvd., Suite 700, Los Angeles, Calif. 90057. *Tel:* (213) 483-3451. Claron L. Oakley, Vice-Pres. and Exec. Ed.

PURPOSE. A nonprofit subsidiary of the California Medical Association, providing continuing education to physicians and hospitals through one-hour subscription tapes of medical meetings and university refresher courses. *Specialization:* continuing education in medicine via audiotapes.
MEMBERSHIP. *Requirements:* must be member of medical or allied professions. *Subscription:* $90/yr. for 24 one-hour recordings (one tape every two weeks).
PUBLICATIONS. Tapes in catalog cover anesthesiology, family practice, internal medicine, ob-gyn, ophthalmology, otorhinolaryngology, pediatrics, psychiatry, and surgery. Payment required with order.

B17. AUDIO-VISUAL ASSOCIATES, 180 E. California Blvd., Pasadena, Calif. 91105. *Tel:* (213) 792-0630. Wesley A. Doak, Owner.

PURPOSE. A consultant firm, providing current information on audiovisual resources via publications, consultation, automation technology, and workshops. *Specialization:* audiovisual consultation.
SPECIAL INFORMATION SERVICES. Audiovisual production and consultation on creation and use of resource centers.
PUBLICATIONS. *International Index to Multi-Media Information* (quarterly), an index to nonbook reviews of bibliographic information. Books and pamphlets on

availability of audiovisual resources, evaluations of in-print materials, planning for resource centers, and staff training. Payment not required with institutional order.

B18. AU-VID, INC., Box 964, Garden Grove, Calif. 92642.* *Tel:* (714) 636-1682.

PURPOSE. To produce audiovisual materials. *Specialization:* self-instruction in medicine.
PUBLICATIONS. Audiovisual series on learning medical terminology, with slides, audiocassettes, and study guides. Large program in audiovascular systems.

B19. A-V SCIENTIFIC AIDS, INC., 639 N. Fairfax Ave., Los Angeles, Calif. 90036.* *Tel:* (213) 658-6911.

PURPOSE. To sell films for patient education and motivation in dentistry and medicine. *Specialization:* patient education.
PUBLICATIONS. Nine films on preventive dentistry (brushing, periodontics, nutrition); five aids (books and audiotapes); ten general-practice films; eleven orthodontic. "Medfact" series of film loops and 35mm filmstrips: cardiovascular, cardiac rehabilitation, ob/gyn, family planning, VD, the eyes, and topics especially for blacks and Hispano-Americans. Payment not required with order.

B20. AVENS (AUDIOVISUAL EDUCATION IN NEUROSURGERY), 15 Columbus Circle, New York, N.Y. 10023. *Tel:* (212) 541-8080. Don Monaco, Program Coord.

PURPOSE. To produce and distribute multimedia packages dealing with neurosurgical techniques. AVENS is an audiovisual journal funded by the Society of Neurological Surgeons Research Foundation, Inc. *Specialization:* neurosurgery.
PUBLICATIONS. Free catalog describes the ten programs now available. Each consists of 30- to 45-minute videocassette playable through standard color TV, illustrated monograph, and set of 34–72 35mm color slides. Series I includes operations on pituitary, cordotomies, and removal of acoustic neuroma. Series II includes intracranial aneurysms, neuralgia, and cervical fusions. Ten-day preview plan available for any one program from which decision can be made on subscribing to one of the series. Each five-unit series priced at $975; individual programs at $300 each.

AYERST LABORATORIES *See* F3

B21. BAKER AND TAYLOR COMPANY, Audiovisual Services Division, Box 230, Momena, Ill. 60954.* *Tel:* (815) 472-2444.

PURPOSE. To supply audiovisual materials.
PUBLICATIONS: Catalog of programs on terminology, nutrition, and fractures. Payment not required with order.

BALTIMORE CITY HEALTH DEPARTMENT *See* D5

B22. BANDERA ENTERPRISES, Box 1107, Studio City, Calif. 91604. *Tel:* (213) 985-5050. Don Flagg, Pres.

PURPOSE. To distribute medical, scientific, and technical films, videotapes, and slides.
PUBLICATIONS. Films, slides, and videotapes. Payment not required with order.

BARTEL DENTAL BOOK COMPANY *See* G13

BAUSCH AND LOMB *See* F4

B23. BAYLOR COLLEGE OF MEDICINE FILM LIBRARY, Texas Medical Center, Houston, Tex. 77025.*

PURPOSE. To produce films for instructional use in medicine. *Specialization:* medical films.
PUBLICATIONS. Many on surgery; large selections in other areas. Catalog available from Baylor; films are for purchase from A-V Corporation, Box 66824, 2518 North Blvd., Houston, Tex. 77006.

B24. R. A. BECKER, INC., Audiovisual Division, 299 Park Ave., New York, N.Y. 10017.*

PURPOSE. To produce audiotapes. *Specialization:* medical audiotapes.
PUBLICATIONS. Taped lectures and symposia for practicing physicians. Each cassette $8.

B25. BECKMAN NEW DIMENSIONS, 3009 S. Daimler St., Santa Ana, Calif. 92705. *Tel:* (714) 556-8560. Ken E. Stine, Mgr.

PURPOSE. To develop, produce, and market technical audiovisual programs and to distribute technical books and manuals. Also offers custom audiovisual program production services.
SPECIAL INFORMATION SERVICES. Custom audiovisual programs.
PUBLICATIONS. "New Dimension" series of audiovisual programs address themselves to 12 scientific areas, including peptide-amino acid analysis, centrifugation, electro-encephalography, electrophoresis, enzymology, and other areas of lab technology used in health sciences. Free catalog provides a detailed and lively listing of available programs. The 40-odd current presentations typically include 30 to 85 color slides, two separate cassette tapes (one for programming slides and one with professional's narration), printed script of all audiomaterial, and an album for filing. "New Dimension" series is an ambitious and professionally packaged product. Worth noting are *Nuclear Medicine Mini-Series* and selections on infrared spectroscopy. Twenty-day preview available. Payment not required with order.
INQUIRY ADDRESS. Beckman New Dimensions, 2500 Harbor Blvd., Fullerton, Calif. 92634. *Tel:* (714) 556-8560.

BECTON-DICKINSON *See* F5.

B26. BEHAVIORAL RESEARCH LABORATORIES, INC., Ladera Professional Center, Box 577, Palo Alto, Calif. 94302.

PURPOSE. To create programmed instruction in reading, math, and science for classroom use. *Specialization:* programmed reading for classrooms.

PUBLICATIONS. Reading materials for programmed instruction in basic biology, health and hygiene, and venereal disease. Thirty-two-page catalog. Payment required with individual order.

B27. BEHAVIORAL SCIENCES TAPE LIBRARY, Sigma Information, Inc., 240 Grand Ave., Leonia, N.J. 07601.

PURPOSE. To distribute and produce audiotapes dealing with behavior. *Specialization:* audiotapes in behavioral sciences.
PUBLICATIONS. Cassettes available in 16 areas, including psychotherapy and psychoanalysis, speech pathology, human sexuality, and feminism. Tapes packaged in boxed sets of 3 to 12 cassettes; also available singly. Payment not required with domestic order.

B28. BELLEFAIRE RESIDENTIAL TREATMENT AND CHILD CARE CENTER, 22001 Fairmount Blvd., Cleveland, Ohio 44118. *Tel:* (216) 932-2800. Laurence A. Grossner, Exec. Dir.

PURPOSE. A residential treatment center for disturbed children. *Specialization:* treatment of mentally disturbed children.
PUBLICATIONS. Two films—*Boy in the Doorway* and *Someday I'll Happy Be.* Rental fee $10. Payment required with order.

B29. BENCHMARK FILMS, INC., 145 Scarborough Rd., Briarcliff Manor, N.Y. 10510. *Tel:* (914) 762-3838.

PURPOSE. To distribute educational films, servicing schools, colleges, and public libraries. *Specialization:* films and filmstrips.
PUBLICATIONS. Films are aimed at school-age audiences, many using humor to make their points. Psychology, behavior, ecology, nutrition, and drug abuse are treated. A treasure trove of Marshall Efron; Efron demonstrates deficiencies in breakfast cereals, frozen lemon pies, and how dolls can stereotype a child's sex roles. Some basic biology films. Also filmstrips. Payment not required with order.

B30. BFA EDUCATIONAL MEDIA, 2211 Michigan Ave., Box 1795, Santa Monica, Calif. 90406. *Tel:* (213) 829-2901. Lloyd Otterman, Gen. Mgr.

PURPOSE. To produce and distribute audiovisual and print educational materials; a division of CBS. (Services restricted to instructors, media coordinators for schools, libraries, training programs, and educational television.) *Specialization:* supplemental educational audiovisual and print materials.
PUBLICATIONS. Films, including documentary film, recently released, exploring careers in health fields. Payment not required with order.

B31. BICOM COMPANY, Box 7233, Pittsburgh, Pa. 15213. *Tel:* (412) 624-3204. David Ross Dickson, Pres.

PURPOSE. To distribute educational materials from research in biocommunications in the form of slides on human anatomy. *Specialization:* slides and prints of human anatomy.

PUBLICATIONS. Catalog lists 14 sets of 35mm color slides, two of which are slide-tape series complete with cassette. (Custom black-and-white prints from any of the slides also supplied.) Some series come with illustrated manual. Concentration on human anatomy—dissections of head, tongue, larynx (mostly of fetuses). Sets cost $25–$266. Ten percent reduction from catalog prices for nonprofit institutions and students. Payment not required with order.

B32. BILLY BUDD FILMS, INC., 235 E. 57 St., New York, N.Y. 10022.*

PURPOSE. To sell and rent 16mm educational films. *Specialization:* maturation and human values.
PUBLICATIONS. Films concerned with growing up, human values, love, sex, death, and dying. Aimed at general audiences.

BIO MONITORING APPLICATIONS, INC. *See* G15

B33. BIOMEDICAL COMMUNICATIONS CENTER—UNIVERSITY OF NE-BRASKA MEDICAL CENTER, 42 and Dewey Ave., Omaha, Nebr. 68105. *Tel:* (402) 541-4304. Reba A. Benschoter, Dir.

PURPOSE. A medical center library engaged in production of audiovisual materials for health science education. *Specialization:* audiovisual materials in medical sciences.
PUBLICATIONS. Films, slides, audiotapes, videotapes, and catalogs. Also 8mm film resource catalog. Payment not required with order.

B34. BLUE HILL EDUCATIONAL SYSTEMS, INC., 120 E. 56 St., New York, N.Y. 10022. *Tel:* (212) 688-2929.*

PURPOSE. To produce instructional videotape programs. *Specialization:* holistic nursing.
PUBLICATIONS. Thirteen 60-minute and nine 30-minute lectures in holistic nursing practices, accompanied by manuals and study guides. Complete *Physical Assessment Course* $3,850. Payment not required with order.

B35. ROBERT J. BRADY COMPANY, The Charles Press, Inc., Bowie, Md. 20715. *Tel:* (301) 262-6300. Robert Brady, Jr., Exec. Vice-Pres.

PURPOSE. To publish multimedia instructional programs. *Specialization:* multimedia instructional programs.
PUBLICATIONS. Texts, films, records, audiotapes, and slides on emergency health care, nursing, elementary/high school instruction in personal health, patient education, crisis intervention, and suicide prevention. Catalog of emergency medical services lists texts in first aid—cardiac arrest, resuscitation, bleeding, and shock, as well as basics of anatomy and terminology. Areas also covered by overhead transparencies, color-sound filmstrips, and 35mm slides. School-age programs feature overhead transparencies that come with instruction guides cover drug abuse, venereal disease, personal health, and information on careers in health. Patient education packages use flipcharts to illustrate nutrition and chronic illnesses. NIMH-sponsored series on crisis intervention uses audiotapes, texts, and films (for purchase)

to present real-life situations in mental care and suicidology. Instructional material in both "high" and "low" lethality situations from attempted suicide to adolescent worries. Medical/Nursing/Allied Health catalog has programs on cardiology, behavioral science, emergencies, programs for allied health assistants, basic therapy, and anatomy. Payment not required with order.

B36. BRIGHAM YOUNG UNIVERSITY, Educational Media Services, 290 HRCB, Provo, Utah 84602. *Tel:* (801) 374-1211, Ext. 2713.

PURPOSE. To rent 16mm films. *Specialization:* educational films.
PUBLICATIONS. Thorough 300-page catalog with detailed descriptions of offerings— alcohol and tobacco, basic and advanced biology, health and hygiene for general audiences, medicine for general audiences, nursing, good mental health practices, dental care. Payment not required with order.

B37. BULLFROG FILMS, INC., Box 114, Milford Square, Pa. 18935.* *Tel:* (215) 536-9060.

PURPOSE. To produce films on world food problems. *Specialization:* nutrition.
PUBLICATIONS. Film, *Diet for a Small Planet*, on organic diets for general audiences. Payment not required with order.

BURGESS PUBLISHING COMPANY *See* G19

BURROUGHS WELLCOME COMPANY *See* F6

CALIFORNIA PEACE OFFICERS' ASSOCIATION *See* A108

CAMPBELL SOUP COMPANY *See* F7

B38. CAMPUS FILM DISTRIBUTORS, 20 E. 46 St., New York, N.Y. 10017. *Tel:* (212) 682-8735. Steve Campus, Pres.

PURPOSE. To distribute educational films. *Specialization:* early childhood education.
PUBLICATIONS. Films emphasize childhood learning, motivation, counseling, reality counseling in New York City schools, children in the hospital, role enactment for children, dramatic play and learning, perceptual learning with blocks, special needs of handicapped children, and play as motivation for learning. Three videotapes on counseling. Aimed at professionals and others involved with counseling or teaching children. For rental or purchase. Payment not required with order.

CANCER CARE, INC. *See* A109

B39. CAREER AIDS, INC., 5024 Lankershim Ave., N. Hollywood, Calif. 91601. *Tel:* (213) 985-5656. Martin W. Early, Pres.

PURPOSE. To produce and distribute training materials in various media for health-care personnel, teachers, and vocational education. *Specialization:* objectives-based training materials.
PUBLICATIONS. Sixteen-page catalog lists multimedia programs, audiocassette pro-grams, and materials in teacher training. Lists level of interest (hospital training,

nursing school, etc.) of programs in ethics, injections, mental health care, geriatrics, and bedside manner. Most are sound-filmstrip combinations, using cassettes or disks at customer's option. Payment not required with order.

B40. CARMAC PRODUCTIONS, 1605 Comanche Trail, Garland, Tex. 75040. *Tel:* (214) 271-1015.*

PURPOSE. To produce evaluation materials for teachers. *Specialization:* education.
PUBLICATIONS. Audiocassette programs on learning needs of all age groups. Includes set on "Mind and Behavior."

CAROLINA BIOLOGICAL SUPPLY COMPANY *See* F9

B41. CAROUSEL FILMS, INC., 1501 Broadway, New York, N.Y. 10036.* *Tel:* (212) BR 9-6734.

PURPOSE. To distribute instructional films for purchase. *Specialization:* sale of instructional films.
PUBLICATIONS. Forty-five-page catalog lists films for sale (Carousel will provide list of distributors that will rent same films, on request)—age level: high school through adult. Health category includes microscopy for general viewers, obesity, air pollution, mental health, a documentary on nursing, CBS-TV's highly acclaimed *Hunger in America* documentary, drugs, basic biology, and human relations. Payment not required with order.

B42. CBS/EDUCATION AND PUBLISHING GROUP, Columbia Broadcasting System, Inc., 383 Madison Ave., New York, N.Y. 10017.* *Tel:* (212) 688-9100. Murray Benson, Vice-Pres.

PURPOSE. A television network offering films to educators through authorized distributors. *Specialization:* educational films.
PUBLICATIONS. Films are copies of CBS-TV broadcasts, listed on 21-page mimeographed guide with appropriate distributors—*Emergency First Aid, Life Before Birth, Atomic Medicine, The Human Heart,* and *The Wild Cell.* Nontechnical presentation; hosts are Walter Cronkite, Roger Mudd, Mike Wallace, and other CBS regulars. Payment is made to particular distributor.

B43. CENTER FOR CASSETTE STUDIES, 8110 Webb Ave., N. Hollywood, Calif. 91605.*

PURPOSE. To produce audiocassettes in psychology. *Specialization:* psychology and psychotherapy.
PUBLICATIONS. Tapes on Gestalt therapy, B. F. Skinner, and psychic healing.

B44. CENTER FOR CONTINUING EDUCATION IN PODIATRIC MEDI-CINE, 148 N. Eighth St., Philadelphia, Pa. 19107. *Tel:* (215) 629-0300. Joel Charles, Dir.

PURPOSE. A consortium of five colleges of podiatric medicine. Produces and distributes audiovisual curriculum and continuing education aids in podiatric

medicine. (Services restricted to medical professionals.) *Specialization:* podiatric
medicine.
SPECIAL INFORMATION SERVICES. One-to-one consultations by specialists on foot
problems for anyone in the medical professions.
PUBLICATIONS. *Audio Journal of Podiatric Medicine* is subscription series of
audiocassettes. *Subscription:* $72.50/yr. for 12 cassettes. Cassettes accompanied by
charts and other illustrative material. Taped seminars and programs for office
assistants as well as practitioners. Surgery, hospital practice, acupuncture, orthopedics, and other areas covered. Books, films, slides, and videotapes available—all for
one-time purchase. Plans are afoot for allowing rental of videocassettes. Payment
required with individual order.

B45. CENTER FOR HUMANITIES, INC., 2 Holland Ave., White Plains, N.Y.
10603.* *Tel:* (914) 946-0601.

PURPOSE. To produce sound-slide programs for classroom use. *Specialization:*
sound-slide programs.
PUBLICATIONS. Catalog worth acquiring for fine reproductions of objets d'art alone.
Illustrations slightly irrelevant, but fun to look at—paintings, sculpture, mixed
media. Actual listings include programs on social and behavioral sciences, personal
development, psychology, health, biology, genetics, and overpopulation. Payment
not required with order.

B46. CENTER FOR MASS COMMUNICATIONS, Columbia University Press,
136 S. Broadway, Irvington, N.Y. 10533.*

PURPOSE. To sell films on health and other topics for general audiences. *Specialization:* educational films.
PUBLICATIONS. Films on the heart, drugs, preventive medicine, environmental
health, venereal disease, importance of health during "the critical decades" (age
40–60), and aging. Payment not required with order.

B47. CENTRE FILMS, INC., 1103 N. El Centro Ave., Hollywood, Calif. 90038.*

PURPOSE. A film distributor. *Specialization:* films.
PUBLICATIONS. *The Story of Eric,* 16mm documentary for sale or rental. Presents
one couple's experiences with birth of their child.

B48. CENTRON EDUCATIONAL FILMS, 1621 W. Ninth St., Lawrence, Kans.
66044. *Tel:* (913) 843-0400. Russell A. Mosser, Pres.

PURPOSE. To produce and market audiovisual materials. *Specialization:* films on
health and safety.
PUBLICATIONS. Catalog of eight color-sound films. Health subjects would appeal to
general audiences. Subjects covered include smoking, unwed pregnancy, jobs in
medicine and health, prenatal care, and venereal disease. Payment required with
order.

B49. CFI—COUNSELOR FILMS, INC., 2100 Locust St., Philadelphia, Pa. 19103.
Tel: (215) 732-9191. Stephen A. Levine, Vice-Pres./Marketing.

PURPOSE. To distribute educational resource material, both audiovisual and printed. *Specialization:* career education and career awareness.
PUBLICATIONS. Colorful catalog of materials on self-awareness and career guidance for elementary and secondary grades. Films and filmstrips explore job options and educational opportunities. Films can be rented or purchased. Also books, videotapes, and audiocassettes. Careers in health fields are covered. Payment not required with order.

CHICAGO COLLEGE OF OSTEOPATHIC MEDICINE—MEDICAL LIBRARY *See* E8

B50. CHURCHILL FILMS, 662 N. Robertson Blvd., Los Angeles, Calif. 90069.* *Tel:* (213) 657-5110. Priscilla Forance, Customer Relations.

PURPOSE. To produce films for the classroom, primary to college levels. *Specialization:* instructional films.
PUBLICATIONS. Thirty-two-page catalog. Films on human body, drugs and alcohol, venereal disease, and safety.

CIBA MEDICAL EDUCATION DIVISION *See* F10

B51. CINEMA CONCEPTS, INC., Middlesex Ave., Chester, Conn. 06412.* *Tel:* (203) 526-9513.

PURPOSE. To produce educational 16mm films. *Specialization:* nutrition.
PUBLICATIONS. "Nutrition A to Z" series—five parts on all aspects of diet for general audiences. Rental or purchase.

B52. CLAY ADAMS, Division of Becton, Dickinson and Company, Parsippany, N.J. 07054.*

PURPOSE. To produce classroom biological training aids. *Specialization:* biology teaching aids.
PUBLICATIONS. Materials are three-dimensional and also graphic. Plastic body parts (torsos, skulls, gestation display), table-top mannequins and slides. Illustrated 65-page catalog. Payment not required with order.

B53. CLEVELAND HEALTH MUSEUM AND EDUCATION CENTER, 8911 Euclid Ave., Cleveland, Ohio 44106. *Tel:* (216) 231-5010. Lowell F. Bernard, Dir.

PURPOSE. To develop effective audiovisual communication programs in health for schools and general public. *Specialization:* health education.
SPECIAL INFORMATION SERVICES. *Special collections:* Dr. Dickenson's original works in sex education.
PUBLICATIONS. Wide range of educational materials for all age groups. Pamphlets, films, slides, audiotapes, videotapes, a newsletter, and three-dimensional exhibits are produced. Good selection of materials on sex education—teaching models, overhead transparencies, 35mm slides, and 16mm film produced for NBC-TV. Also materials on anatomy, venereal disease, dental care, dangers of smoking, and drug abuse. Periodicals available only to members. Payment required for some audiovisual orders and all orders for exhibits.

COLLEGE OF AMERICAN PATHOLOGISTS *See* A114

B54. COLLEGE OF SAINT TERESA, Audio Visual Center, Winona, Minnesota.*
Sister Irma Recker, Dir., Audiovisual Aids.

PURPOSE. To produce series of films for training nurses.
PUBLICATIONS. Four films cover general care, intravenous feeding, and food.
Handling fee $4. Payment required with order.

B55. COMMUNICATION SKILLS CORPORATION, 1220 Post Rd., Box 684,
Fairfield, Conn. 06430.* *Tel:* (203) 255-5944.

PURPOSE. To produce multimedia teaching aids. *Specialization:* instructional audiovisual materials.
PUBLICATIONS. Programs on lab technique, biochemistry, spectroscopy, allied
health, and food technology skills. For high school and more advanced levels.

B56. COMMUNICATIONS IN LEARNING, INC., 2929 Main St., Buffalo, N.Y.
14214.* *Tel:* (716) 837-7555.

PURPOSE. To produce audiovisuals for teaching. *Specialization:* audiotape slide
programs.
PUBLICATIONS. Audiotape slide programs include a number aimed at health practitioners for training. Series includes management of health-care facilities, clinical
pastoral education, occupational therapy, physical therapy, dentistry, nursing,
medicine, hospital librarianship, and others. Most lectures are between $9 to $20.
Previews available for a fee. Payment required with order.

B57. CONCEPT MEDIA, 1500 Adams Ave., Costa Mesa, Calif. 92626.* *Tel:* (714)
549-3347.

PURPOSE. To produce multimedia teaching programs for nurses. *Specialization:*
nursing.
PUBLICATIONS. Filmstrip-audiocassette-manual combinations cover "The Stroke
Patient," "Nurse-Patient Interaction," "Perspectives on Dying," "Pain/Sleep,"
"Fundamentals of Nursing," and "Cancer" (three series).

B58. CONCORDIA AUDIOVISUAL MEDIA, 3558 S. Jefferson Ave., St. Louis,
Mo. 63118.*

PURPOSE. A distributor of contemporary materials for Christian education and
information. *Specialization:* audiovisual materials.
PUBLICATIONS. Eighty-page catalog of various media. Rental and sale films on
alcohol, drugs, marriage and the family, and sex education. Religious, highly
moralistic slant. Also records and cassettes. Payment not required with order.

B59. CONRAD BERENS INTERNATIONAL EYE FILM LIBRARY, INC., 246
Danforth Ave., Jersey City, N.J. 07305. *Tel:* (201) 332-6685. Patricia Rainier,
Admin.

PURPOSE. To provide audiovisual medical teaching material to professionals in ophthalmology. (Services not available to lay groups.) *Specialization:* ophthalmology and allied subjects.
PUBLICATIONS. Twenty-four-page catalog listing approximately 90 films; additional 20 in supplement. All are technical explorations of anatomy of eyes, eye surgery, etc. Payment not required with order.

B60. CONTINUING EDUCATION IN NEUROLOGICAL SCIENCES, 25 E. Washington, Chicago, Ill. 60602.*

PURPOSE. To produce lectures in neurology on audiotape. *Specialization:* neurological sciences.
PUBLICATIONS. Neurological sciences lectures presented at Cook County Graduate School of Medicine, February 1975. Complete set (84 cassettes) $386.40. Also, attache case for $28.00. Payment not required with order.

COOK-WAITE LABORATORIES *See* F11

B61. CORNELL UNIVERSITY EDUCATIONAL TELEVISION CENTER, New York State College of Human Ecology, Martha van Rensselaer Hall, Ithaca, N.Y. 14850.* *Tel:* (607) 256-5431.

PURPOSE. To rent and sell videotapes and 16mm films. *Specialization:* educational TV programs on tape.
PUBLICATIONS. Eighteen-page list. Distribution of some productions is restricted. TV stations in New York State may use them free of charge. Human development and family studies, nutrition, aging, drugs, and sexuality. Payment not required with order.

B62. CORONET INSTRUCTIONAL MATERIALS, 65 E. South Water St., Chicago, Ill. 60601.*

PURPOSE. To produce audiovisuals for purchase. *Specialization:* instructional audiovisual programs.
PUBLICATIONS. Sound filmstrips, study prints, 8mm loops, audiocassettes, and multimedia units. Health materials for primary level (hygiene, diet, exercise). Basic biology and ecology for high schools, jobs in health services (sound filmstrip series), and other topics. Payment not required with order.

B63. CREATIVE LEARNING CENTER, 105 Edgevale Rd., Baltimore, Md. 21210.* *Tel:* (301) 532-6357.

PURPOSE. To produce audiovisual materials for classroom use. *Specialization:* instructional audiovisual productions.
PUBLICATIONS. Films for purchase or rental on natural childbirth, nontraditional marriages, drugs, sickle-cell anemia, tuberculosis, and lead poisoning. Audiocassettes on birth control, venereal disease, and alcohol. Payment not required with order.

CREIGHTON UNIVERSITY HEALTH SCIENCES LIBRARY *See* E11

B64. CRM PRODUCTIONS, Marketing Department, 9263 W. Third St., Beverly Hills, Calif. 90210.* *Tel:* (213) 273-4930.

PURPOSE. To produce and distribute *Psychology Today* films. *Specialization:* films on psychology.
PUBLICATIONS. CRM is the organization that publishes *Psychology Today* (monthly), a psychology review for the general reading public emphasizing social psychology and behavior. Same emphasis evident in films listed in catalog: series on behavior modification features talks with dean of behavioral school, Dr. B. F. Skinner. Also has film on application of behavior modification to business, specifically Emery Air Freight and that company's experiences with Skinnerian technique in use on employees. Other films deal with sensation and learning, development, social psychology, and personality. A 97-page *Film Guide* expounds on use of films in classroom. Material aimed at college level and professionals in behavioral sciences. Six life science documentaries planned (cells, evolution, muscles, heart, and sensory world to be covered). Payment not required with order.

B65. CURRICULUM MATERIALS CORPORATION, 1319 Vine St., Philadelphia, Pa. 19107.* *Tel:* (215) MA7-4600.

PURPOSE. To produce sound-filmstrips for school-age audiences (grades K-4). *Specialization:* primary level filmstrips.
PUBLICATIONS. Filmstrips on hygiene, anatomy, dental care, and diet; series on "Your Body" and "Health Habits." Payment not required with order.

B66. DATAFILMS, 2625 Temple St., Los Angeles, Calif. 90026. *Tel:* (213) 385-3911. Mrs. Iona Harrison, Print Mgr.

PURPOSE. To rent and sell films and videotapes. *Specialization:* educational films.
PUBLICATIONS. 16mm films (produced by Parthenon Pictures), super-8 cartridges, and videocassettes. Contact-lens use and care, planned parenthood for the poor, social need for population control, and series of eight films on safety.

B67. DAVIDSON FILMS, INC., 3701 Buchanan St., San Francisco, Calif. 94123.* *Tel:* (415) 567-2974.

PURPOSE. To produce and sell 16mm educational films. *Specialization:* educational films.
PUBLICATIONS. Series of four on Piaget's developmental theory for students in psychology, education, child development, and other areas. Payment not required with order.

F. A. DAVIS COMPANY *See* G24

B68. DAYTON LAB, 3235 Dayton Ave., Lorain, Ohio 44055.*

PURPOSE. To publish guide to multimedia programs for learning medicine. *Specialization:* medical instructional programs.
PUBLICATIONS. Listing of individualized learning materials in medicine. Detailed

subject listing of 4,000 programs in all media, arranged by titles with subject index and list of producers. Payment not required with order.

DEFENSE CIVIL PREPAREDNESS AGENCY *See* D8

DENAR CORPORATION *See* F12

B69. DENOYER-GEPPERT AUDIO-VISUALS, 355 Lexington Ave., New York, N.Y. 10017. *Tel:* (212) 682-1600. Howard H. Rosenheim, Pres.

PURPOSE. To produce educational audiovisual materials. *Specialization:* instructional audiovisuals.
PUBLICATIONS. Thirty-page science catalog of films, filmstrips, sound filmstrips, overhead transparencies, film loops, and slides. Aimed at high school/college audiences. Large selection in biology, chemistry, and general science. Separate 45-page elementary/junior high catalog on health and hygiene, venereal disease, and psychology handled in similar media. Thirty-two-page medical and biological sciences catalog featuring classroom charts, slides, and three-dimensional plastic displays of organs, skeletal system, and reproductive system. Payment not required with order.
INQUIRY ADDRESS. 5235 Ravenswood Ave., Chicago, Ill. *Tel:* (312) 561-9200.

DEVEREUX FOUNDATION *See* A119

B70. A. B. DICK AUDIO VISUAL OPERATIONS, 5950 W. Touhy Ave., Chicago, Ill. 60648.*

PURPOSE. A manufacturer of copying machines, office equipment, and audiovisual projectors and support equipment. Also produces films and film loops. *Specialization:* instructional audiovisuals.
PUBLICATIONS. Catalog lists 2,000 super-8mm film loops (for A. B. Dick model 60 projector or equivalent) and their distributors. Health, family life education (conception, birth, sexuality) are dealt with (for school-age audiences), plus basic biology and life sciences. Most loops for primary to high school levels. Catalog comes with order cards.

B71. DIRECTION SOUTH MEDIA, Hunt Valley, Md. 21031.* *Tel:* (301) 666-7778.

PURPOSE. To produce audiovisual programs for professionals. *Specialization:* sound-filmstrips for medical professionals.
PUBLICATIONS. Available filmstrip-audiocassette programs illustrate methods for examining patients and surgical procedures; includes *A Method for Suction Curettage.* $30/program.

B72. DOCUMATIC FILMS, INC., 5 Andover Rd., Hartsdale, N.Y. 10530.* *Tel:* (914) 428-3568.

PURPOSE. A film producer. *Specialization:* films.
SPECIAL INFORMATION SERVICES. *Languages:* English and Spanish.

PUBLICATIONS. A film *A Family Is Born*, for families expecting a child, illustrating various delivery methods. Preview available. Purchase price $250.

DRUG INTELLIGENCE PUBLICATIONS *See* G28

B73. DRUSTAR, INC., 1385 Brookham Dr., Grove City, Ohio 43123.*

PURPOSE. To rent and sell audiovisual training programs. *Specialization:* programs for training medical personnel.
PUBLICATIONS. Series on "Nurse's Aide In-Service Training" (film cassettes or videotapes), includes projection equipment. Purchase price $1,250; rental $114.37 for 12 lessons.

B74. DUKANE CORPORATION, Audio-Visual Division, 2900 Dukane Dr., St. Charles, Ill. 60174.*

PURPOSE. To produce software for audiovisual systems. *Specialization:* audiovisual products.
PUBLICATIONS. List of producers (not titles) of sound-filmstrips and number of titles they carry on given subjects, including health and safety.

B75. DUKE UNIVERSITY MEDICAL CENTER, Division of Audiovisual Education, Durham, N.C. 27710.*

PURPOSE. To produce and sell audiovisual programs for teaching health professionals. *Specialization:* audiovisual instruction in health.
PUBLICATIONS. Catalog lists offerings, with abstract of each program, indexes by subject and format. Most for instruction of health professionals, some for patient education. Well-produced and informative catalog; all programs produced at Duke.
INQUIRY ADDRESS. Director, Division of Audiovisual Education, Box 3163, Duke University, Durham, N.C. 27710.

EATON MEDICAL FILM LIBRARY *See* F14

B76. EDCOA PRODUCTIONS, INC., 520 S. Dean St., Englewood, N.J. 07631.*
Tel: (201) 567-0820 or (212) 721-2100.

PURPOSE. To produce films for professionals. (Films on human sexuality restricted to professionals and accredited institutions or social agencies.) *Specialization:* human sexuality.
PUBLICATIONS *Relax and Enjoy It*, a film for patient counseling. For rent or purchase.

EDUCATIONAL FOUNDATION OF THE AMERICAN SOCIETY OF PLASTIC AND RECONSTRUCTIVE SURGEONS, INC. *See* A122.

B77. EDUCATIONAL INNOVATORS PRESS, Box 13052, Tucson, Ariz. 85732.*

PURPOSE. To produce sound-filmstrip programs for educators. *Specialization:* audiovisual instruction for educators.

PUBLICATIONS. Filmstrip-audiocassette combinations on student-management and behavior. Seven programs on behavior, including psychomotor behavior.

B78. EDUCATIONAL PERSPECTIVES ASSOCIATES, Box 213, DeKalb, Ill. 60115.*

PURPOSE. To produce audiovisual programs in patient care and other areas. *Specialization:* sound-filmstrips for instruction.
PUBLICATIONS. Filmstrip-audiocassette programs on death, geared to elementary level. Teacher guides also available. Strips sold in packages or individually.

B79. EDUCATIONAL PRODUCTS INC., 5005 W. 110 St., Oak Lawn, Ill. 60453.* *Tel:* (312) 425-0800.

PURPOSE. A service of Westinghouse Learning Corporation, producing audiovisual programs for training and instructing medical professionals. *Specialization:* instructional programs in medicine.
PUBLICATIONS. Mixed-media programs on patient care and basic medical sciences. Twenty-seven learning modules titled *Health Instructional Programs for Professionals* (HIPP) and Ohio State University *Independent Study Program in Medicine* (ISP). Previews available.

B80. EDUCATIONAL PROJECTIONS CORPORATION, 3070 Lake Terrace, Glenview, Ill. 60025.* *Tel:* (312) 729-4200. Lora Cook, Dir. of Instructional Materials.

PURPOSE. To produce filmstrip programs. *Specialization:* filmstrips.
PUBLICATIONS. List of dealers of EPC materials, which are geared to primary grades and cover health and safety in such areas as first aid, anatomy, personal hygiene, and physical fitness. Some accompanied by audiocassettes.

B81. EDUCATIONAL RESOURCES FOUNDATION, 2712 Millwood Ave., Columbia, S.C. 29250.* *Tel:* (803) 253-3389.

PURPOSE. To produce audiovisual materials. *Specialization:* multimedia instructional programs.
PUBLICATIONS. Slide-tape programs, including series of six on "Stroke: How to Care," geared to nurses and others responsible for patient care, accompanied by script. Series $240.

B82. EDUCATIONAL TV—COMMUNICATIONS OFFICE FOR RESEARCH AND TEACHING, University of California, San Francisco, Calif. 94143. *Tel:* (415) 666-1958. Thomas L. Banks, Coord.

PURPOSE. To provide continuing education video materials for health professionals. *Specialization:* general medicine, pediatrics, ob/gyn, psychiatry, radiology, and neurology.
PUBLICATIONS. Four postgraduate videotape training programs in radiology; six approaches to brief psychotherapy; Grand Rounds (televised seminars) in medicine, neurology, obstetrics/gynecology, pediatrics, psychiatry, and surgery. Videotapes

can be ordered in Ampex 1", ½", or ¾" videocassette. 16mm film on self-help for women on reaching orgasm, for use in sex education and training, clients of counselors and researchers. Payment required with order.

EDUCATORS PROGRESS SERVICE, INC. *See* G29

B83. EMCOM, INC., 4000 W. 76 St., Minneapolis, Minn. 55435.*
PURPOSE. To produce audiovisual programs. *Specialization:* alcoholism.
PUBLICATIONS. *The Caring Community*, videocassette and film series on alcoholism and drug dependence. Developed in cooperation with Hazelden Rehabilitation Center.

EMPLOYERS INSURANCE OF WAUSAU *See* F15

B84. ENCYCLOPAEDIA BRITANNICA EDUCATIONAL CORPORATION, 425 N. Michigan Ave., Chicago, Ill. 60611. *Tel:* (312) 321-7000. Ralph Wagner, Exec. Vice-Pres. for Marketing.
PURPOSE. To produce and distribute audiovisual and other educational materials. *Specialization:* educational films and filmstrips.
SPECIAL INFORMATION SERVICES. *Languages:* English and Spanish.
PUBLICATIONS. Exciting, well-produced 160-page film catalog. Films are for general, mostly school-age audiences; include biology, ecology, human life, general health and hygiene, diseases, nutrition, and fitness—many available in Spanish. 8- or 16mm film or videocassettes. Can be rented or purchased. Color-illustrated 100-page catalog of filmstrips, kits, books, study prints, records, slides, and 8mm films on life science, animal life, human life, and chemistry, as well as general health and safety. Payment not required with order.
INQUIRY ADDRESS. Robert Brown, Instructional and Library Services, 425 N. Michigan Ave., Chicago, Ill. 60611. *Tel:* (321) 312-7320.

EPILEPSY FOUNDATION OF AMERICA *See* A124

EXCERPTA MEDICA B.V. *See* G31

B85. EYE GATE HOUSE, 146-01 Archer Ave., Jamaica, N.Y. 11435. *Tel:* (212) 291-9100. Robert F. Newman, Pres.
PURPOSE. To produce audiovisual educational materials. *Specialization:* filmstrips on health for schools.
PUBLICATIONS. Large, color-illustrated catalog of over 3,600 filmstrip, loop, and transparency titles, levels K–college. Health instruction covers first aid, venereal disease, diet, nutrition, exercise, alcoholism, sexuality, and drug abuse; biology, anatomy, and physiology for school-age audiences. Filmstrips with disc or cassette soundtracks, 8mm silent loops, and overhead transparencies. Previews available, and free Quickstrips showing filmstrips printed out, with narration. Payment not required with order.

B86. FAIRCHILD CAMERA AND INSTRUMENT CORPORATION, 75 Mall Dr., Commack, N.Y. 11725.* *Tel:* (516) 864-8500.

PURPOSE. To manufacture specialized photographic systems for education, industry, and science. *Specialization:* audiovisual hardware.
PUBLICATIONS. Catalog contains subject listing of films and their distributors. Fairchild will assist in locating films by subject if not listed in catalog, those grouped together under medicine number in the hundreds, with no further breakdown on specific areas.

B87. FARM FILM FOUNDATION, Southern Building, Suite 424, 1425 H St. N.W., Washington, D.C. 20005. Charles E. Palm, Pres.

PURPOSE. A nonprofit institution for creating better understanding between rural and urban America through audiovisual education. *Specialization:* agricultural films.
PUBLICATIONS. 16mm sound films, including some on nutrition. Free to groups.

FEDERAL AVIATION ADMINISTRATION *See* D9

B88. FILMMAKERS LIBRARY, INC., 290 West End Ave., New York, N.Y. 10023.*

PURPOSE. To produce motion pictures. *Specialization:* educational films.
PUBLICATIONS. Films on birth and death, some having been shown on national public television. Rentals and preview available.

B89. FLORIDA STATE UNIVERSITY MEDIA RENTAL LIBRARY Instructional Media Center, Division of Instructional Research and Service, Florida State University, Tallahassee, Fla. 32306. *Tel:* (904) 644-2820. Dan Isaacs, Dir.

PURPOSE. Rental of instructional films.
SPECIAL INFORMATION SERVICES. *Languages:* English, French, German, Spanish, and Russian.
PUBLICATIONS. 465-page catalog gives description, age level, and other information. Selections in health sciences emphasize personal hygiene, nutrition, and medicine for general audiences. Wide variety on many topics. Rental. Payment not required with order.

FOOD AND DRUG ADMINISTRATION *See* D10

B90. FOUNDATION FOR LIVING, Abbott-Northwestern Hospital Corporation, Chicago Ave. at 27 St., Minneapolis, Minn. 55407.*

PURPOSE. To produce audiovisual programs on alcoholism. *Specialization:* alcoholic rehabilitation.
PUBLICATIONS. Films and audiocassettes on rehabilitation of alcoholics. Six programs in all. Payment required with order.

B91. FRANCISCAN FILMS, Box 6116, San Francisco, Calif. 94101.*

PURPOSE. To produce films.
PUBLICATIONS. Brochure describes *You Got What?*, a 16mm color and sound film, which, according to the description, is an awareness film on venereal disease. For

secondary and above levels. A preview print is available without charge. Purchase price $275; daily rental $25; weekly rental $50.

GASP (GROUP AGAINST SMOG AND POLLUTION) *See* A127

GEIGY PHARMACEUTICALS *See* F16

B92. GEORGIA REGIONAL MEDICAL TELEVISION NETWORK, A. W. Calhoun Medical Library, Woodruff Memorial Building, Emory University, Atlanta, Ga. 30322.*

PURPOSE. A circulating library of videocassettes.
PUBLICATIONS. Member teaching institutions can borrow tapes free or purchase at 25 percent discount. Nonmembers pay fee for borrowing or full price for purchase. Carefully selected professional-level programs of high quality, covering all medical specialties. Programs number about 250.

B93. GLENN EDUCATIONAL MEDICAL SERVICES, INC., Box 381, Monsey, N.Y. 10952.* *Tel:* (212) 292-8159.

PURPOSE. To produce audiovisual instructional programs in medicine. *Specialization:* audiovisual programs in respiratory therapy.
PUBLICATIONS. Overhead transparencies, slides, and workbooks in "coordinated learning systems" for practitioners and medical students. Beginning and advanced respiratory therapy. Payment not required with order.

B94. GRAPHIC FILMS CORPORATION, 3341 Cahuenga Blvd. W., Hollywood, Calif. 90028.*

PURPOSE. To produce films. *Specialization:* medical films.
PUBLICATIONS. Productions aimed at professionals. *Embryology and Pathology of the Intestinal Tract,* for purchase; preview available.

B95. GREAT PLAINS NATIONAL INSTRUCTIONAL TELEVISION LIBRARY, Box 80669, Lincoln, Nebr. 68501.*

PURPOSE. A network for distribution of videocassettes and films. *Specialization:* audiovisual programs for general audiences.
PUBLICATIONS. Materials are for rent generally and some can be purchased. Some free previews possible. Elementary through college levels, plus adult. Health areas include public health, science, mental health, and dental health. Catalog.

B96. GUIDANCE ASSOCIATES, 757 Third Ave., New York, N.Y. 10017. *Tel:* (212) 754-3700. John H. Fisher, Pres.

PURPOSE. A division of Harcourt Brace Jovanovich, producing instructional media for grades K–14. *Specialization:* instructional films and filmstrips on personal health and adolescent psychology for school-age audiences.
PUBLICATIONS. Catalogs describe available films and sound filmstrips. Nutrition series features three-part filmstrip program on food values, psychology of eating, and

basic food groups. Other programs on smoking, drinking, family living, and problems of adolescence. Venereal disease filmstrips for different age levels. Catalogs contain useful information on how to effectively organize media instruction. Sound tracks can be on either discs or tape cassettes. Also eight 16mm color films on growth and family life. Programs can be viewed on approval. Payment not required with order.

B97. HALLMARK FILMS AND RECORDINGS, INC., Educational Division, 1511 E. North Ave., Baltimore, Md. 21213. *Tel:* (301) 837-3516. Max Brecher, Pres.

PURPOSE. To produce audiovisual material in field of special education. *Specialization:* sex education and behavior modification.
PUBLICATIONS. Films on alternatives to traditional marriage, sex education, behavior modification, early childhood learning, and teaching skills to mentally retarded. Also slides and videotapes. Payment not required with order from accredited purchasers.

HARPER AND ROW PUBLISHERS *See* G34

B98. HARRIS-TUCHMAN PRODUCTIONS, INC., 751 N. Highland Ave., Hollywood, Calif. 90038.* *Tel:* (213) 936-7189.

PURPOSE. To produce sound-filmstrips. *Specialization:* audiovisual programs for medical instruction.
PUBLICATIONS. Filmstrips come with audiocassettes, include series on defibrillators and pacemakers, legal aspects of nursing, others for hospital staffs and M.D.s. Free previews. For rent or purchase.

HARVARD UNIVERSITY PRESS *See* G35

B99. HEALTH EDUCATION AIDS, 8 S. Lakeview, Goddard, Kans. 67052.

PURPOSE. To produce multimedia programs. *Specialization:* health instruction.
PUBLICATIONS. Sets of filmstrips accompanied by audiocassettes and booklets— basic anatomy, physiology, and nursing. Free previews.

B100. HEALTH EDUCATION PROGRAMS, INC., 65 E. 55 St., New York, N.Y. 10022.*

PURPOSE. To produce audiovisual programs in health. *Specialization:* emergency management.
PUBLICATIONS. Series on emergency management, which uses HEP's own special viewing equipment. Format called "visual cassette"; viewer comes with series or separately.

B101. HEALTH MANAGEMENT SYSTEMS INC., 1455 Broad St., Bloomfield, N.J. 07003.* *Tel:* (201) 338-3615.

PURPOSE. To produce modular audiovisual systems. *Specialization:* health-care management and administration.

PUBLICATIONS. System contains audiocassette and text. Of special interest is the TIME (Techniques to Improve Management Efficiency) system.

HILTZ AND HAYES PUBLISHING COMPANY, INC. *See* G37

B102. HEALTH SCIENCES COMMUNICATION CENTER, Case Western Reserve University, 2119 Abington Rd., Cleveland, Ohio 44106. *Tel:* 368-3776. William T. Stickley, Dir.

PURPOSE. To provide and acquire all forms of nonprint materials for instructional programs of schools of dentistry, medicine, and nursing. (Services restricted to personnel in health sciences.) *Specialization:* medical films and videotapes.
PUBLICATIONS. Ten-page dentistry catalog. Videotapes and slide/tapes on prostheses, instruments, and handling child patients. Brochures on individual health productions: videotaped instruction on continuous flow liquid analyzer; film on use of nasal CPAP; slide set on ocular fundus; film meant to prepare children for surgery; film/videotape on evaluating infant maturity; others. Payment not required with order.

B103. HOSPITAL RESEARCH AND EDUCATIONAL TRUST, 840 N. Lake Shore Dr., Chicago, Ill. 60611.*

PURPOSE. To provide informative audiotapes for hospital trustees. *Specialization:* hospital trusteeship.
PUBLICATIONS. Audiocassettes include *A Trustee Talks with Trustees, Health Care Trends,* and similar topics. Tapes $20–$40. Payment required with order.

HOWARD UNIVERSITY—MEDICAL-DENTAL LIBRARY *See* E18

B104. INSIGHT FILMS—PAULIST PRODUCTIONS, 17575 Pacific Coast Hwy., Pacific Palisades, Calif. 90272.* *Tel:* (213) 454-0688. Richard Welch, Exec. Dir. of Education.

PURPOSE. To present dramatizations on film of crucial problems facing young people. *Specialization:* filmed dramatizations dealing with problems of youth.
PUBLICATIONS. Ten-page illustrated catalog. Films seem to take nondenominational slant, are professionally produced, and not to be considered propaganda for Paulists. Originally produced for the highly acclaimed *Insight* TV series on Sunday-morning broadcasts, films boast stars such as Howard Duff, Brian Keith, Harvey Korman, and Jane Wyatt. *Exit* and *The Sandalmaker* deal realistically with drugs, giving no pat, simplistic answers; *The Party* deals in same manner with sex. 16mm with sound. For sale or rent. Payment not required with order.

B105. INSTRUCTIONAL DYNAMICS, INC., 450 E. Ohio St., Chicago, Ill. 60611. *Tel:* (312) 943-1200. Dr. Philip Lewis, Pres.

PURPOSE. To develop and distribute materials dealing with human development and interpersonal communications. *Specialization:* audiotapes in human relations.
PUBLICATIONS. Twenty-five-page catalog. Experiences in interpersonal relations, encounter group material, marriage counseling, Carl Rogers, minority training

programs, transactional analysis, and raising children. Concentration on self-discovery and personal awareness; instructions for professionals in analysis and encounter. Payment required with individual order.

B106. INTERNATIONAL FILM BUREAU, INC., 332 S. Michigan Ave., Chicago, Ill. 60604. *Tel:* (312) 427-4545.

PURPOSE. To produce and distribute educational films and filmstrips. *Specialization:* films and filmstrips.
SPECIAL INFORMATION SERVICES. *Languages:* English and Spanish.
PUBLICATIONS. Materials are aimed at general audiences. Health and welfare catalog lists films and filmstrips on aging, child care, mental health, drug and alcohol abuse, history of medicine, nursing, and other topics. Films can be purchased or rented from IFB or rented from regional agents. Separate brochure lists films on mental health, delinquency, ethics, counseling, growing up, and family life. Also list of new films with some in health field. Some with Spanish track. Payment not required with order.

JASON ARONSON, INC. *See* G40.

B107. JERI PRODUCTIONS, Box 693, Big Bear City, Calif. 92314. Geraldine Jensen, Producer/Owner.

PURPOSE. To publish record albums in health education and physical education. *Specialization:* speech, relaxation, and body improvement.
PUBLICATIONS. Instructive phono records aimed at elementary grades, but also useful in remedial speech classes at all levels. Learn proper sitting with Posture Paul, learn how to relax, and how to smile with the Happy Clown and the Sad Clown. "Say and Sing" series teaches pronunciation. Eleven different albums listed. Payment not required with order.

B108. THE JOHNS HOPKINS UNIVERSITY PRESS—AUDIO-VISUAL DIVISION, 3400 Charles St., Baltimore, Md. 21218. *Tel:* (301) 366-9600, exts. 57 and 58. John R. Riina, Mgr., Audio-Visual Div.

PURPOSE. To publish scholarly audiovisual materials. *Specialization:* medicine.
PUBLICATIONS. Audiovisual materials for the medical professions with emphasis on continuing medical education programs for physicians. Books, pamphlets, slides, and audiotapes. Payment not required with order.

JOHNSON ASSOCIATES *See* G42

JOHNSON AND JOHNSON *See* F17

KANSAS STATE UNIVERSITY—VETERINARY MEDICAL LIBRARY *See* E24

B109. LAWREN PRODUCTIONS, INC., Box 1542, 1881 Rollins Rd., Suite C, Burlingame, Calif. 94010. *Tel:* (415) 697-2558. Thomas G. Gregory, Exec. Vice-Pres.

PURPOSE. To produce and distribute film and TV programs. *Specialization:* medically oriented film production.
PUBLICATIONS. Folders describe various films available for rental and purchase. Lawren distributes California Medical Association film library productions, mainly clinical studies aimed at professionals, detailing diagnoses and treatments. Some CMA films aimed at lay viewers. Films on mental illness, learning disabilities, adolescent growth, unwed motherhood, and childbirth will appeal to wide audience. Dangers of smoking treated in serious movies and in a farcical look at tobacco industry's power called *Too Tough to Care.* Payment not required with order.

B110. LEARNING CORPORATION OF AMERICA, 711 Fifth Ave., New York, N.Y. 10022.* *Tel:* (212) 751-4400.

PURPOSE. A subsidiary of Columbia Pictures, distributing films for educators' use, including guidance films. *Specialization:* films on learning and guidance.
PUBLICATIONS. Fifty-five-page catalog lists short films on pollution and effects on humans. Guidance films are segments of feature releases, starring Jack Nicholson, Nichol Williamson, and others, accompanied by teacher's guide to leading discussion on subjects like identity, conformity, etc. Aimed at junior-senior high school and college-adult levels. For rent or purchase. Payment not required with order.

LEARNING DYNAMICS, INC. *See* G45

LIBRARY OF CONGRESS CATALOG PUBLICATION DIVISION *See* D12

ELI LILLY AND COMPANY *See* F18

B111. LISTENING LIBRARY, INC., One Park Ave., Old Greenwich, Conn. 06870.* A. Ditlow, Pres.

PURPOSE. To distribute multimedia instructional materials to educators. *Specialization:* instructional materials for the classroom.
PUBLICATIONS. One-hundred-twenty-eight-page catalog of phono records, audiocassettes, and filmstrips for all grade levels. Topics include health and safety, personal development, physical education, sex, drug abuse, personal hygiene, and fundamentals of biology. Payment required with individual order.

B112. MACMILLAN FILMS, 34 MacQuesten Parkway S., Mt. Vernon, N.Y. 10550. *Tel:* (914) 664-4277. Myron Bresnick, Pres.

PURPOSE. To sell and rent 16mm films. *Specialization:* educational films.
PUBLICATIONS. Well-illustrated, provocative 235-page catalog. Varied selections from many sources, such as the TV networks, colleges, museums, and foreign producers. Health topics (for general audiences) include alcohol and other drugs, tobacco use, psychology (with interview series featuring Skinner, Rogers, and other noted psychologists), biology, public health, and mental illness. New features on acupuncture, euthanasia, the food industry, and child abuse; Joe Namath warns about danger of injuries in sports. Payment not required with order.

MEDICAL EXAMINATION PUBLISHING COMPANY, INC. *See* G48

B113. McGRAW-HILL FILMS, 1221 Ave. of the Americas, New York, N.Y. 10020. *Tel:* (212) 997-4409. Alan Kellock, Vice-Pres. and Gen. Mgr.

PURPOSE. To produce and distribute films, sound filmstrips, and multimedia packages. *Specialization:* instructional audiovisuals for general audiences.
PUBLICATIONS. Separate catalogs for instructional films; audiovisuals for grades K–12. Catalogs are attractive, professionally produced guides to materials. Films cover education, careers, guidance, and health—all intended for general public. Age levels elementary school to adult. Impressive selection of 16mm films from National Film Board of Canada, TV networks, McGraw-Hill. Also feature films such as *Panic in Needle Park*, with Al Pacino; Leni Riefenstahl's *Olympia*, and *Free to Be/You and Me*. Health films on venereal disease, drinking, smoking, and adolescent psychology. Filmstrips for grades K–6 cover dental care, nutrition, and hygiene; grades 7–12 strips concentrate on career guidance, science, and social studies. Some available as 8mm silent loop or with sound on record or tape cassette. Payment not required with order.

B114. THE MEDICAL MEDIA NETWORK, University Extension, University of California, 10995 LeConte Ave., Room 540, Los Angeles, Calif. 90024. *Tel:* (213) 825-7781. Jan MacAlister, Distr. Mgr.

PURPOSE. To distribute audiovisual programs (film and videotape) for use in continuing education for physicians and in in-service training of allied health personnel. *Specialization:* audiovisual programs in medicine and allied health professions.
PUBLICATIONS. *Medical Media: An Approach to Learning* is a lively, professional, coherent guide to use of audiovisuals in health fields. Describes in orderly fashion how to identify learning needs, preview available media, incorporate the media into the existing teaching program, and stimulate motivation to learn. Is intended for use with "Medical Media Network" series, but lessons contained can be applied to use of audiovisuals in general. A "utilization manual" that would be valuable for anyone concerned with incorporating audiovisual education into existing learning framework.
Medical Media Network itself consists of some 40 programs, most available as Jayark super-8mm cartridges, Ampex 1″ videotapes, and 16mm films. Catalog gives complete rundown on subject, intended audience (physicians, nurses, planners, etc.), and faculty involved. Largest selections are on internal medicine and nursing. Special film on utilization of MMN programs can be used free of charge for two weeks. Programs for rent or purchase. Payment required with order.

B115. MEDICAL UNIVERSITY OF SOUTH CAROLINA—DEPARTMENT OF AUDIOVISUAL RESOURCES, Charleston, S.C. 29401. *Tel:* (803) 792-3001. Stephen P. Dittmann, Chmn., DAVR.

PURPOSE. To provide wide variety of audiovisual production and consultation services and instructional design for faculty and staff of Medical University. (Services restricted to faculty and staff of MUSC. Special consideration given at times to contractual agreements for production for clients outside university.) *Specialization:* medical audiovisual productions.

PUBLICATIONS. Films, slides and audio- and videotapes produced by DAVR may be available from faculty member or department for whom developed. Titles numerous and varied.

B116. MEDICAL UNIVERSITY OF SOUTH CAROLINA—DIVISION OF CONTINUING EDUCATION/HEALTH COMMUNICATIONS NETWORK, 16 Bee St., Charleston, S.C. 29401. *Tel:* (803) 792-4241. Dr. Vince Moseley, Dir.

PURPOSE. To provide continuing education for all professional and nonprofessional personnel in 25 hospitals in South Carolina. Also produces open circuit programs for lay audience for airing over ETV in South Carolina. (Certain subject matter, mainly psychiatry, restricted to member hospitals or Medical University.) *Specialization:* continuing education in medicine.

MEMBERSHIP. South Carolina hospitals pay dues as part of network membership; materials available to other agencies at stated costs.

SPECIAL INFORMATION SERVICES. *Special collections:* ROCOM Help series, ROCOM Intensive Coronary Care course, NCME subscription and special order, Pharmacy series, Heaton series, and Management of Patient Account services.

PUBLICATIONS. Two catalogs, one covering audiocassettes and one videocassettes, list offerings. Tapes of symposia and seminars, along with taped lectures. Videotapes, mostly in color, are described in catalog as to hosts and content. Hundreds of selections. Payment required with order.

B117. MENTAL HEALTH TRAINING FILM PROGRAM, 33 Fenwood Rd., Boston, Mass. 02115. *Tel:* (617) 566-6793. Edward A. Mason, M.D., Dir.

PURPOSE. A film producer attached to Harvard Medical School, distributing educational films in areas of mental health and health education. *Specialization:* mental health.

PUBLICATIONS. Listing of films on preventive intervention, classroom challenges; "Camp Wediko" series explores problems and behavior of emotionally disturbed boys at therapeutic summer camp in New Hampshire. Other topics include underachievement, consultation, and history of psychiatry. Payment not required with order.

MICHIGAN CANCER FOUNDATION *See* A147

MICROCARD EDITIONS *See* G49

B118. MILNER-FENWICK INC., Educational Division, 3800 Liberty Heights Ave., Baltimore, Md. 21215.

PURPOSE. To distribute audiovisual materials in health and other areas of instruction. *Specialization:* films and multimedia programs.

PUBLICATIONS. Films and slide programs—home dental care, clinical courses in dental assisting, advances in human genetics, patient counseling, human sexuality, diabetes, emergency treatment, and more. Largest section of films is on genetics. Payment not required with order.

B119. MODERN TALKING PICTURE SERVICE, 2323 New Hyde Park Rd., New Hyde Park, N.Y. 11040. *Tel:* (516) 437-6300. Carl H. Lenz, Pres.

PURPOSE. To distribute motion pictures and videocassettes. *Specialization:* free-loan films and videotapes.
PUBLICATIONS. 16mm sound/color films loaned to nontheatrical business and industry, school, community and adult groups, and TV stations. Free-loan 35mm shorts to theaters. Health-related topics include nutrition, personal hygiene, and growing up. Films are produced by corporations, government agencies, and other associations. Films from Exxon, California Prune Advisory Board, U.S. Army, Baha'i Faith, J. C. Penney, Mrs. Smith's Pie Company, etc. Several programs on ¾" videocassettes.

B120. MOUNTAIN PLAINS EDUCATIONAL MEDIA COUNCIL, c/o University of Wyoming, Audiovisual Services, Laramie, Wyo. 82070. *Tel:* (307) 766-3184.

PURPOSE. A coordinating center for 16mm educational films held by members— universities of Colorado, Nevada, Wyoming, and Utah.
PUBLICATIONS. Over 600-page film catalog. Films are rented from four cooperating centers. Aimed at general audiences—first aid and hygiene, along with general information on diseases covered, along with titles in health careers and nursing. Large selection in biology, a few in psychology. Good choice of titles in genetics and heredity, microbiology, natural history, and human zoology (anatomy). Payment not required with order.

NATIONAL AGRICULTURAL LIBRARY *See* D14

NATIONAL ASSOCIATION FOR MENTAL HEALTH, INC. *See* A150

NATIONAL ASSOCIATION FOR MUSIC THERAPY *See* A151

NATIONAL ASSOCIATION OF BLUE SHIELD PLANS *See* A154

NATIONAL AUDIOVISUAL CENTER *See* D15

B121. NATIONAL CENTER FOR AUDIO TAPES, 364 Stadium Building, University of Colorado, Boulder, Colo. 80302. *Tel:* (303) 492-7341. Robert W. Bruns, Supvr.

PURPOSE. To serve as repository of noncopyrighted educational audiotape programs, duplicating them on order from nonprofit levels, and increasing collection through production and exchange. *Specialization:* noncopyrighted audiotapes.
PUBLICATIONS. Catalog ($4.50) lists 14,000 audio programs in humanities and sciences. Purchasers of tapes may make unlimited copies. In health, 144 programs; diseases, 70; and 93 in general medicine. Tapes aimed more at general audiences than practicing professionals introduce diseases and treatments, health and hygiene, drugs, careers in medicine, and other topics. $2.40–$2.90 each. Payment required with order.

B122. NATIONAL FILM BOARD OF CANADA, 1251 Ave. of the Americas, New York, N.Y. 10020.* *Tel:* (212) 586-2400. John Boundy, U.S. Gen. Mgr.

PURPOSE. To produce and sponsor films, underwritten by government of Canada. *Specialization:* films in health, growing up, psychology, and other areas.
PUBLICATIONS. One-hundred-and-twenty-page catalog lists films available through distributors for rental or sale. (Board does not distribute its own films to public.) Many are rented through McGraw-Hill Films. Guide is well produced and gives descriptions of current Film Board offerings. In health and medicine, aimed at both professional and general viewers, board offers animated films on conception and contraception, pros and cons of smoking, venereal disease, dental problems, diet, menstruation, and film biography of Canadian physician Dr. Norman Bethune, hero of Spanish Civil War and Chinese Revolution. "Child Development" series looks at the terrible twos, frustrating fours, and their siblings of different ages. Good selection in mental health and safety, biology, and ecology. National Film Board of Canada has been acclaimed many times and has received many international cinema awards for its productions. It offers wide variety and high quality to user of instructional films; studios in Montreal produce over 100 films yearly.

NATIONAL FOUNDATION FOR SUDDEN INFANT DEATH *See* A165

NATIONAL FOUNDATION—THE MARCH OF DIMES *See* A166

NATIONAL MEDICAL AUDIOVISUAL CENTER *See* D21

NATIONAL PUBLIC RELATIONS COUNCIL OF HEALTH AND WEL-FARE SERVICES *See* A171

NATIONAL SAFETY COUNCIL *See* A173

NEW YORK STATE HEALTH DEPARTMENT *See* D22

B123. NEW YORK UNIVERSITY FILM LIBRARY, 26 Washington Place, New York, N.Y. 10003. *Tel:* (212) 598-2250. Dr. Daniel Lesser, Dir.

PURPOSE. The acquisition and distribution of 16mm educational, scientific, and documentary films to educational institutions, industries, community agencies, and organized groups. *Specialization:* teacher education and behavioral sciences.
PUBLICATIONS. Catalogs. Payment not required with order.

NORTH CAROLINA SAFETY CONFERENCE *See* A175

PROSTHETIC-ORTHOTIC CENTER—NORTHWESTERN UNIVERSITY *See* H10

B124. NUTRITION SERIES, 311-0 E. Sierra Madre Blvd., Sierra Madre, Calif. 91024. *Tel:* (213) 355-9186. Charles Bish, D.D.S., Owner.

PURPOSE. To produce and distribute dental health programs on filmstrips and records. (Services restricted to schools and government health departments.) *Specialization:* dental health.

PUBLICATIONS. Sound filmstrips *How the Royal Family Learned to Be Happy* (dental care and nutrition for preschool and kindergarten) and *Cutters, Tearers, Crushers and Grinders* (same topics, for grades 1–3). Payment required with orders for previews.
INQUIRY ADDRESS. Charles Bish, Suite 106, 75 N. Santa Anita Ave., Arcadia, Calif. 91006. *Tel:* (213) 445-2726.

B125. OHIO STATE UNIVERSITY—DEPARTMENT OF PHOTOGRAPHY AND CINEMA, 156 W. 19 Ave., Columbus, Ohio 43215. *Tel:* (614) 422-5966. George D. Barber, Film Distribution Supvr.

PURPOSE. To produce 16mm educational sound films. *Specialization:* educational and medical films.
PUBLICATIONS. Twenty-page illustrated catalog. Over 50 titles in medicine— anatomy, surgery, eye care, nutrition, rehabilitation, child development, and diagnosis; about 20 titles in nursing. Medical films for both professionals and laymen; also filmstrips. Payment not required with order.

OHIO STATE UNIVERSITY PHARMACY LIBRARY *See* E32

B126. ORTHOPAEDIC AUDIO-SYNOPSIS FOUNDATION, 1510 Oxley St., Suite B, South Pasadena, Calif. 91030. *Tel:* (213) 682-1760. Alice Harris, Managing Ed.

PURPOSE. To provide educational services for orthopedic surgeons in training and in practice. *Specialization:* orthopedic surgery.
PUBLICATIONS. Audiocassettes, issued on monthly basis, are aimed at practicing orthopedic surgeons. Orthopedists describe various diagnoses and treatments. Large selection described in two brochures. Subscription $75.

B127. OXFORD FILMS, INC., 1136 N. Las Palmas Ave., Los Angeles, Calif. 90038, *Tel:* (213) 461-9231. Martin Kleiman, Pres.

PURPOSE. A subsidiary of Paramount Pictures, distributing educational 16mm films in health and other related areas. *Specialization:* educational films.
Special Information Services. *Languages:* English, French, and Spanish.
PUBLICATIONS. Eighty-page catalog of almost 400 films, with illustrations and detailed descriptions of each offering. Aimed at elementary through secondary school audiences, this covers health and hygiene, venereal diseases, family planning, biology, drugs and alcohol, and other topics. Payment not required with order.

B128. PARENTS' MAGAZINE FILMS, INC., 52 Vanderbilt Ave., New York, N.Y. 10017, *Tel:* (212) 685-4400, ext. 225. Thaomas Sand, Vice-Pres.

PURPOSE. To produce audiovisual materials for furthering understanding of the child's physical and mental development and of the complexities in marriage and family living. *Specialization:* child behavior, development, and health; parenthood; pregnancy; prenatal care; marriage and family living.
PUBLICATIONS. Sound filmstrips on moral development in children, child development and child health, marriage, pregnancy, childbirth, child behavior, and under-

standing parenthood. 16mm film on development of feelings in children. Other materials on nutrition, love, economics, and other topics. All are explained in colorful illustrated folders. Payment not required with order.

B129. PARSONS STATE HOSPITAL—MEDIA SUPPORT SERVICES, Parsons, Kans. 67357. *Tel:* (316) 421-6550, ext. 234. Howard U. Bair, M.D., Supt. and Medical Dir.

PURPOSE. To prepare training materials for those concerned with the developmentally disabled. *Specialization:* media production.
PUBLICATIONS. Books, pamphlets, films, slides, audio- and videotapes. Includes catalog of films available through Kansas Center for Mental Retardation and Human Development at Lawrence. These films cover therapy for the retarded, counseling, physical difficulties, and drugs. Some films rented free. Payment not required with order.

B130. PARTHENON PICTURES/DATAFILMS, 2625 Temple St., Los Angeles, Calif. 90026. *Tel:* (213) 385-3911. Charles Palmer, Exec. Producer.

PURPOSE. To distribute educational and documentary films. *Specialization:* employee training and occupational safety.
PUBLICATIONS. *Wheelchair Driver-Training* for patients and attendants; films on pharmacy, pharmaceutical research, planned parenthood, and population control. Super-8 cartridges, 16mm, and videocassettes. Some films free-loan. Payment not required with order.

B131. PERENNIAL EDUCATION, INC., 1825 Willow Rd., Northfield, Ill. 60093.* *Tel:* (312) 446-4153.

PURPOSE. To provide sound-filmstrips and films for classroom use. *Specialization:* audiovisual materials on family living.
PUBLICATIONS. Materials cover sex education for primary through high school levels (plus some for parents), family planning, venereal diseases, childbirth, sex and the handicapped, and transvestitism and lesbianism. Also drugs and drinking and their effects. One-volume guide to materials in mental health and family-life education for teachers, educators, and librarians—$35. Payment not required with order.

PERSONAL PRODUCTS COMPANY *See* F20

B132. PHYSIOLOGICAL TRAINING COMPANY, 2485 Huntington Dr., San Marino, Calif. 91108.* *Tel:* (213) 793-9149.

PURPOSE. To sell audiovisual materials and equipment for medical training. *Specialization:* medical training systems.
PUBLICATIONS. Offerings in audiovisual programs incude TUTOR Arrhythmia Recognition Training System, programmed tapes that play heartbeats over cardioscopes. Accompanied by taped narration. Payment not required with order.

PLANNED PARENTHOOD FEDERATION OF AMERICA *See* A184

B133. POLYMORPH FILMS, 331 Newbury St., Boston, Mass. 02115.* *Tel:* (617) 262-5960.

PURPOSE. To produce educational films for general audiences. *Specialization:* educational films.
PUBLICATIONS. For rental and purchase, Polymorph offers films on preparation for childbirth (Lamaze method in particular), breastfeeding, and mentally retarded children. Payment not required with order.

PRENTICE-HALL *See* G54

B134. PRIMARY MEDICAL COMMUNICATIONS, 122 E. 42 St., New York, N.Y. 10017.*

PURPOSE. To distribute videocassettes for physicians and other medical professionals. Some aimed at lay audiences. *Specialization:* videotape cassettes. Payment not required with order.

PRINCETON MICROFILM CORPORATION *See* G55

B135. PROFESSIONAL ARTS, INC., Box 8003, Stanford, Calif. 94305. *Tel:* (415) 365-6630. Norman MacLeod, Pres.

PURPOSE. Specialists in film and audio communications. *Specialization:* traffic safety and drug education.

B136. PROFESSIONAL INFORMATION LIBRARY, 1616 HiLine Dr., Dallas, Tex. 75207. *Tel:* (214) 747-2537. Bertram S. Resnick, Exec. Producer/Ed.

PURPOSE. To produce audio- and videotape cassettes in medical specialties and special-order patient education programs. *Specialization:* neurosurgery, neurology, pharmacology, historical medicine, forensics, medical-legal problems, and medical socioeconomic problems.
PUBLICATIONS. Taped journals, incorporating highlights of conferences and symposia, and reviews of printed journals, such as *New England Journal of Medicine.* Audio journals include *Neurosurgery Review, Neurology Review, Audio Drug News,* and *Historical Reflections.* Slides and videotapes on medical subjects. Payment required with videotape orders.

B137. PROFESSIONAL RESEARCH, INC. 660 S. Bonnie Brae, Los Angeles, Calif. 90057. *Tel:* (213) 483–6220. Dr. Norman Traverse, Pres.

PURPOSE. To produce and distribute patient-counseling films. (Services restricted to hospitals, physicians, and universities.) *Specialization:* films on health care.
PUBLICATIONS. Pamphlets, films, and videotapes. Films for counseling patients on chronic diseases and on self-examination; also dentistry, general hygiene, and eye care. Also films for continuing education. Illustrated, professionally produced catalog. Super-8mm continuous-loop cartridges. Payment not required with order.

B138. PSYCHODYNAMIC RESEARCH CORPORATION, Englewood, N.J. 07632.*

PURPOSE. To produce educational programs on audiocassettes. *Specialization:* audiocassettes on psychology and related topics.

PUBLICATIONS. Tapes concerned with alcoholism, drugs, suicide prevention, crisis intervention, and psychological afflictions (manic-depressives, schizophrenics, anxiety-prone). Payment required with individual order.

B139. PSYCHOLOGICAL CINEMA REGISTER—PENNSYLVANIA STATE UNIVERSITY, Audio-Visual Services, 17 Willard Building, University Park, Pa. 16802. *Tel:* (814) 865-6315. T. M. Reeves, Head, Audio Visual Services.

PURPOSE. A specialized collection of rental and sales films in the behavioral sciences, designed to fill instructional needs and to document original research. *Specialization:* psychology, psychiatry, behavior, and anthropology.

PUBLICATIONS. Annotated 140-page catalog, available at no charge, gives descriptions of all films and is a very helpful guide to choosing films to order. Largest selections are in animal behavior, childhood/development, ethnology, psychopathology, and therapy. All films are in 16mm, most have sound, some are in color.

PAYMENT. Catalog free, reissued about every three years; all films listed can be rented, some purchased. Payment not required with order; preview prints can be obtained if a film is being seriously considered for purchase. NOTE: some films are restricted as to showings and can be rented for teaching, clinical, or conference purposes.

SPECIAL COLLECTION. Encyclopedia Cinematographica, with films depicting single phenomena or types of behavior. Penn State Audio-Visual Services also provides catalogs of materials in biology, chemistry, and physics.

B140. PSYCHOLOGICAL FILMS, INC., 1215 E. Chapman Ave., Orange, Calif. 92666. *Tel:* (714) 639-4646.

PURPOSE. To produce 16mm films in psychology. *Specialization:* films on psychology.

PUBLICATIONS. Attractive and innovative catalog with descriptions of each film and illustrations. Films on encounter, Gestalt, actualization, sex roles, childhood, starring Carl Rogers, Rollo May, Fritz Perls, and Viktor Frankl. Twenty films listed for rent or purchase—all 16mm, some also on videocassettes. Payment not required with order.

PUBLIC AFFAIRS COMMITTEE *See* A188

B141. PUBLIC TELEVISION LIBRARY, Public Broadcasting Service, 475 L'Enfant Plaza S.W., Washington, D.C. 20024.* *Tel:* (202) 488-5000.

PURPOSE. To rent and sell TV programs produced by PBS. *Specialization:* videotaped PBS broadcasts.

PUBLICATIONS. Sixty-five-page, well-produced and informative catalog. Programs were nationally televised productions, some put together by PBS member stations (WGBH, Boston; WNET, New York; KQED, San Francisco, etc.); others produced by PBS. Topics examined include unwed pregnant women, drug abuse, autistic children, mongolism, vasectomies, health-care delivery in rural areas (in this case,

Tennessee), smoking, alcoholism, and series of 30 half-hour programs on human sexuality. Payment not required with order.

B142. PYRAMID FILMS, Box 1048, Santa Monica, Calif. 90406.* *Tel:* (213) 828-7577. David Adams, Pres.

PURPOSE. To sell and rent 16mm films. *Specialization:* instructional films.
PUBLICATIONS. Hefty, professional-looking catalog of 242 pages, detailing descriptions of offerings. Available as 16mm, super 8mm, or videocassette. Includes *The Chemical Man* (biochemistry for everyone), as well as dozens of others of interest to school-age and general audiences—first aid, smoking, the heart, acupuncture, alcohol, safety, ecology, sex, etc. Payment not required with order.

B143. Q-ED PRODUCTIONS, Box 1608, 2921 W. Alameda Ave., Burbank, Calif. 91507.* *Tel:* (213) 848-6637. Edward D. Eagle, Pres.

PURPOSE. To sell filmstrips for primary grades through high school. *Specialization:* filmstrips for classroom use.
SPECIAL INFORMATION SERVICES. *Languages:* English and Spanish.
PUBLICATIONS. Filmstrips treat use of drugs, nutrition, sex, growing up, and similar topics for classroom viewers. Payment not required with order.

REHABILITATION INSTITUTE OF CHICAGO *See* H11

REHABILITATION INTERNATIONAL, USA *See* A190.

B144. RESCUE BREATHING FILM ASSOCIATES, 10505 Hillhaven, Tujunga, Calif. 91042. *Tel:* (213) 352-4661.

PURPOSE. To produce and distribute films on emergency first aid and rescue. *Specialization:* emergency first-aid treatment.
PUBLICATIONS. Films demonstrating rescue breathing for victims of suffocation by shock, drowning, drugs, and other emergencies. Film on emergency treatment of heart attack victims. Book on producing educational films. Films and book described in brochures. Payment not required with order.

B145. RESEARCH MEDIA, INC., 4 Midland Ave., Hicksville, N.Y. 11801. *Tel:* (516) 433-5672. Leonard Louis, Pres.

PURPOSE. To produce and distribute multimedia instructional programs. *Specialization:* multimedia instructive programs.
PUBLICATIONS. Catalogs of programs in nursing and allied health sciences, behavior modification training, and introduction to psychology. First covers physiology, technical nursing concepts, and radiology for use in nursing schools, hospitals, and other schools for training nurses, lab technicians, paramedics, etc. Also includes patient education and medical self-instruction courses. Materials on behavior modification and introductory psychology rely on slide/tape programs for self-instruction in these areas. Payment not required with order.

B146. RMI EDUCATIONAL FILMS, INC.—WESTWOOD EDUCATIONAL PRODUCTIONS, 701 Westport Rd. Kansas City, Mo. 64111.* *Tel:* (816) 561-2285.

PURPOSE. To sell educational films for school-age audiences. *Specialization:* educational films.
PUBLICATIONS. Topics include human sexuality and basic biology. Payment not required with order.

A. H. ROBINS COMPANY *See* F21

ROCHE FILM LIBRARY *See* F22

ROERIG DIVISION FILM LIBRARY *See* F24

ROSS AUDIO VISUAL LIBRARY *See* F25

B147. ST. LUKE'S HOSPITAL, 2900 W. Oklahoma Ave., Milwaukee, Wisc. 53215.* *Tel:* (414) 647-6423. Jack Ellingboe, AV Coord.

PURPOSE. A hospital with videotape library, renting tapes for showings to professionals. *Specialization:* medical videotapes.
PUBLICATIONS. Three-page mimeo list. Rent $10/week—1″ Ampex VTR and ¾″ U-Matic cartridges. Payment not required with order.

SANDOZ PHARMACEUTICALS *See* F26

B148. SATURN SCIENTIFIC, INC., Box 2417, 540 Northeast Eighth St., Fort Lauderdale, Fla. 33303.*

PURPOSE. To provide visual aids for professional audiences. *Specialization:* medical visual aids.
PUBLICATIONS. Supplies of transparencies and microsections in biology, anatomy, histology, and pathology for use by professionals, medical students, and institutions. *Introduction to Human Anatomy* (192 color slides with script); *Biology of Reproduction* (150 slides with script); microsections and photomicrographs of human and some animal tissues. Blood and marrow smears, bacteria, and parasites on microslides. Seventy-page catalog. Minimum order $10. Payment not required with order.

SCHERING PROFESSIONAL FILM LIBRARY *See* F27

B149. SCHLOAT PRODUCTIONS, 150 White Plains Rd., Tarrytown, N.Y. 10591.* *Tel:* (914) 631-8300.

PURPOSE. To produce instructional media for schools. *Specialization:* filmstrips for the classroom.
PUBLICATIONS. Color sound-filmstrips on reproduction, human physiology, other areas of biology (most for high school and college levels), and biochemistry. Illustrated catalog. Payment not required with order.

B150. W. SCHWANN, INC., 137 Newbury St., Boston, Mass. 02116.*

PURPOSE. To publish guides to current records and tapes. *Specialization:* listings of newly released records and audiotapes.
PUBLICATIONS. *Schwann 2* (semiannual supplement to *Schwann 1,* the pop, rock, and classical listings) lists instructional records and tapes with prices. Schwann is

considered the Bible of the purchaser of newly released tapes and discs. $1/vol. Payment required with order.

SCIENCE AND HEALTH PUBLICATIONS *See* G62

B151. SCIENTIFICOM—LARUE COMMUNICATIONS, 708 N. Dearborn, Chicago, Ill. 60610. *Tel:* (312) 787-8656. Gunter H. Doetsch, Pres.

PURPOSE. To produce motion pictures and to distribute audiovisual material for the health-care field. (Service restricted to health-care professionals.) *Specialization:* medical and scientific audiovisuals.
SPECIAL INFORMATION SERVICES. *Languages:* English, French, Spanish, Portuguese, and Creole (Haitian).
PUBLICATIONS. Catalog and press releases describe scientific film inventory. Majority are 16mm films produced by hospitals, professional organizations, medical schools, and pharmaceutical companies. Includes series of 12 films on trauma produced by American College of Surgeons. Films listed can be rented or purchased; some titles provided free for viewing by producers. Free-loan productions include ones on heart attack prevention, streptococcal disease control, and venous cutdowns. Majority of films on surgery and operating room technique; some on personal health for general audiences. Catalog describes films as to content and audience recommended (professional, school-age, etc.). Slide presentations are also listed. Payment required with order for rent or preview if credit not established.

G. D. SEARLE AND COMPANY *See* F28

SHELL FILM LIBRARY   F29

SIGNAL PRESS *See* G63

B152. SISTER KENNY INSTITUTE, 1800 Chicago Ave., Minneapolis, Minn. 55404. *Tel:* (612) 871-7331. Dr. L. Leslie, Pres.

PURPOSE. A rehabilitation institute involved in patient care, continuing education, and publications and audiovisual materials. *Specialization:* long-term care nursing, rehabilitation, and special learning.
PUBLICATIONS. Booklets on physical therapy, ambulation, stroke, guides for nurses, choosing wheelchairs, colostomy, and ileostomy. Slide programs, mostly on care of disabled. Audiocassettes on native American values versus white culture's; other topics similar to booklets; five films on patient care, several others on stroke. Filmstrips. Payment required with order of less than $10.

SMART FAMILY FOUNDATION *See* A192

SMITH, KLINE, AND FRENCH *See* F30

B153. SMITH, MILLER AND PATCH, INC., 401 Joyce Kilmer Ave., New Brunswick, N.J. 08901.*

PURPOSE. A free-loan film library for medical professionals. *Specialization:* films for professionals.
PUBLICATIONS. Seventy-five-page list of films on ophthalmology.

SOCIETY FOR RESEARCH IN CHILD DEVELOPMENT, INC. *See* A194.

B154. SOCIETY FOR VISUAL EDUCATION, INC., 1345 Diversey Parkway, Chicago, Ill. 60614. *Tel:* (312) 525-1500, WATS (800) 621-1900. Charles F. Keffer, Pres.

PURPOSE. A division of Singer, producing audiovisual materials. *Specialization:* audiovisual materials.
PUBLICATIONS. Sound and captioned filmstrips, slides, records, audiotapes, 8mm film loops, learning modules and study prints, and overhead transparencies. Personal health and hygiene, sex education, drug abuse, venereal disease, diet and nutrition, mental health are covered. Materials aimed at school-age audiences. Payment required with individual order.

B155. SOUNDWORDS, INC., 56-11 217 St., Bayside, N.Y. 11364.*

PURPOSE. To produce audiocassettes on health information for the general public. *Specialization:* audiocassettes on health.
PUBLICATIONS. Cassettes are nontechnical presentations by doctors on sexuality, diabetes, hay fever, lung diseases, obesity, and cardiac problems. Intended for use by industry, schools, libraries, medical institutions, and community and other groups. Eighteen titles. Payment not required with order.

B156. SOUTHERN ILLINOIS UNIVERSITY, Learning Resources Service, Carbondale, Ill. 62901.*

PURPOSE. To rent films on health for general audiences. *Specialization:* health films.
PUBLICATIONS. Films are on obesity, maternity care, alcoholism, first aid, psychology, and nutrition. Mimeographed list of titles. Payment not required with order.

SOUTHERN MEDICAL ASSOCIATION *See* A197

SPECTRUM PUBLICATIONS, INC. *See* G67

B157. SPENCO MEDICAL CORPORATION, Box 8113, Waco, Texas 76710.*
Tel: (800) 433-2400 (from outside Texas only).

PURPOSE. To produce visual aids and printed material on dangers to health, morality, and the public good. *Specialization:* audiovisual productions on health.
PUBLICATIONS. Posters and displays warn against smoking, drinking, etc. Sample slogans: "Ban the Butt," "Virtue Won't Hurt You," "Smut Smells," "Acid Heads Are Hollow." Less alarmist family-planning display (mounted loops, pills, and condoms) and mounted lung, artery, and tooth specimens. "Health Insight" audiocassette library on breast care, venereal disease, obesity, and common health issues. Buttons, games, balloons. *Alive and Well* (bi-monthly), $5.95/yr., carries articles by physicians on common health problems. Payment not required with order.

SQUIBB MEDICAL FILMS *See* F31

B158. STANTON FILMS, 7934 Santa Monica Blvd., Los Angeles, Calif. 90046. *Tel:* (213) 656-8656. Thomas J. Stanton, Owner.

PURPOSE. To produce and distribute educational films. *Specialization:* educational films.
PUBLICATIONS. Five 16mm color films, 10 minutes each. Aimed at younger children, they concern exercise, sleep and rest, nutrition, eyesight, and personal hygiene. Purchase $125 each. Payment not required with order.

STATE OF CALIFORNIA DEPT. OF HEALTH *See* D27.

STATE OF MAINE DEPT. OF HEALTH AND WELFARE *See* D28.

B159. STERLING EDUCATIONAL FILMS, 241 E. 34 St., New York, N.Y. 10016. *Tel:* (212) 683-6300. Leonard Feldman, Vice-Pres.

PURPOSE. To distribute films to educational market. *Specialization:* educational films.
PUBLICATIONS. Films, aimed at school-age audiences, include personal health, dental care, venereal disease, and sexuality. Eighty-page catalog is lively and well illustrated. Films are mainly intended for purchase. Payment not required with order.

B160. STUART FINLEY, INC., Department R, 3428 Mansfield Rd., Falls Church, Va. 22041.* *Tel:* (703) 820-7700.

PURPOSE. To distribute films for general audiences. *Specialization:* educational films.
PUBLICATIONS. Topics include ecology and retarded children (*Becky* and four other films are on retardation). Payment not required with order.

B161. STUART REYNOLDS PRODUCTIONS, INC., 9465 Wilshire Blvd., Beverly Hills, Calif. 90212. *Tel:* (213) 274-7863. Stuart Reynolds, Pres.

PURPOSE. To produce and distribute 16mm educational films. *Specialization:* educational films.
SPECIAL INFORMATION SERVICES. *Languages:* English, French, and Spanish.
PUBLICATIONS. *The Eye of the Beholder,* a film examining perception, human relations, and transactional analysis. Recommended by producer for classes in psychology, social psychiatry, and psychiatric nursing. Payment not required with order.

B162. SUNBURST COMMUNICATIONS, Fancher Rd., Pound Ridge, N.Y. 10576.* *Tel:* (914) 764-5737. Warren Schloat, Pres.

PURPOSE. To produce films and sound-filmstrips for classroom use. *Specialization:* films for school-age audiences.
PUBLICATIONS. Productions, aimed generally at high school level, cover marriage, first aid, nutrition, venereal disease, drugs, and dying. Payment not required with order.

SUNKIST GROWERS, INC. *See* F32

SYNTEX LABORATORIES, INC. *See* F33

B163. TEACH 'EM, INC., Department C-2, 625 N. Michigan Ave., Chicago, Ill. 60611.* Aaron Cohodes, Pres.

PURPOSE. To distribute audiotapes on health. *Specialization:* health-care management and administration.

PUBLICATIONS. Audiocassettes, listed in 30-page catalog, stress management practices, medical staff administration, emergency care, and patient education. Cassettes accompanied by study guides and reprints. Payment not required with order.

B164. TEACHING FILMS, INC., Division of A-V Corporation, 2518 North Blvd., Box 66824, Houston, Tex. 77006. *Tel:* (713) 523-6701. J. C. Rebman, Pres.

PURPOSE. To produce and distribute motion pictures on health sciences for use in medical schools. *Specialization:* films on human anatomy.

PUBLICATIONS. Catalog lists six series of films on anatomy: 20 films in dissection, illustrating gross anatomy; 42 on more specific regions; 7 on human eye; 20 on anatomical basis of brain function; 26 on skeletal and topographic anatomy; and large series in production on histology. Some series come with study guides for class use. Previews available; films are for purchase. Payment not required with order.

B165. TELEPHONE LECTURE NETWORK, 2929 Main St., Buffalo, N.Y. 14214. *Tel:* (716) 835-0728.

PURPOSE. To prepare lectures in health care and related services for continuing education and in-service training. Lectures developed in cooperation with leading health institutions, agencies, and organizations in New York and Pennsylvania. *Specialization:* health care and public health.

PUBLICATIONS. Basis of system is prerecorded audiocassettes, often accompanied by 35mm slides, charts, graphs, bibliographies, and other printed materials. Catalogs (based on computer printouts) are offered in dentistry, medicine and surgery, nursing, podiatry, and allied health areas. Latter catalog covers food service, medical librarianship, therapy, and other fields. Catalogs are thorough, giving summaries of lectures and descriptions of accompanying materials. Payment required with order.

B166. TELSTAR PRODUCTIONS, 366 N. Prior, St. Paul, Minn. 55104. *Tel:* (612) 644-4726. Dr. Victor Kerns, Gen. Manager.

PURPOSE. To produce and distribute instructional video programs. *Specialization:* nursing education and communications skills.

PUBLICATIONS. Seventy-five-page catalog of videotaped programs on anatomy and physiology, history of nursing and nursing in society, microbiology, pharmacology, and psychology. Several dozen half-hour programs in each area. Smaller catalog of video instructional materials includes psychology and personal growth. Different formats of tapes available. Payment not required with order.

B167. TEMPLE UNIVERSITY HEALTH SCIENCES CENTER, Department of Medical Communications, 3400 N. Broad St., Philadelphia, Pa. 19140.* Stanton W. Saltzman, Dept. Dir.

PURPOSE. To maintain audiovisual collection for use at Temple Health Sciences Center. *Specialization:* audiovisual collection in health sciences.
PUBLICATIONS. Two-hundred-page index of holdings—videotapes, films, slides, and audiotapes for medical school instruction. Requests for off-campus use should be directed to department director.

C. S. TEPFER PUBLISHING COMPANY, INC. *See* G73

B168. TEXAS WOMEN'S UNIVERSITY—COLLEGE OF NURSING, Educational Television Project, 1130 M. D. Anderson Blvd., Houston, Tex. 77025.* Edith Wright, R.N., Proj. Dir.

PURPOSE. To produce and distribute videotapes. *Specialization:* videotapes for nurses' training in public health.
PUBLICATIONS. "Public Health Science for Baccalaureate Nursing Programs," a series of 30 half-hour lessons, with teacher's guide for each lesson; for institutions training nurses. Payment not required with order.

B169. THREE-M COMPANY, Visual Products Division, 3M Center, St. Paul, Minn. 55101.*

PURPOSE. To produce raw materials for audiovisual use, as well as finished overhead transparencies. *Specialization:* overhead transparencies and supplies.
PUBLICATIONS. Prepared overhead transparencies and masters for classroom use, grades K–12. Hygiene, nutrition, and growth covered, and an interesting selection on community health. Payment not required with order.

B170. TIME-LIFE FILMS, 1271 Ave. of the Americas, New York, N.Y. 10020.* *Tel:* (212) JU 6-1212. Bruce L. Paisner, Pres.

PURPOSE. To produce instructional films for primary grades through adult levels. *Specialization:* instructional films for the classroom.
SPECIAL INFORMATION SERVICES. *Languages:* English and Spanish.
PUBLICATIONS. One-hundred-page illustrated *Multimedia Educational Resources Catalog,* well produced and informative. Films and videotapes listed can be purchased or rented; cover biology, drug problems, and pollution. Good psychology selection. Payment not required with order.

B171. TUFTS UNIVERSITY MEDICAL SCHOOL—EDUCATIONAL MEDIA CENTER, 136 Harrison Ave., Boston, Mass. 02108. *Tel:* (617) 423-4600, ext. 264. Mary B. Allen, Dir.

PURPOSE. To produce teaching aids. *Specialization:* videotape production for student instruction, continuing education, and patient care.
SPECIAL INFORMATION SERVICES. Source information on data retrieval and consultation on teaching materials.

PUBLICATIONS. Videotapes, slide/tape packages, photography, films. Catalog being prepared. Payment not required with order.

UNIPUB *See* G75

B172. UNIVERSAL EDUCATION AND VISUAL ARTS, 221 Park Ave. S., New York, N.Y. 10003.*

PURPOSE. To distribute films for primary through college levels and for teacher education. *Specialization:* audiovisual aids for classroom use.
PUBLICATIONS. Film catalog and catalog for multimedia (sound filmstrips and silent super-8, loops, and transparencies). Childbirth film for high school and college viewers, physical education, ecology, and basic biology in animals and humans. Payment not required with order.

B173. UNIVERSITY OF ALABAMA SCHOOL OF DENTISTRY, University Station, Birmingham, Ala. 35294.*

PURPOSE. To produce audiovisual programs for dental professionals. *Specialization:* dentistry.
PUBLICATIONS. *Four-Handed Dentistry Manual,* $6. Five 16mm films, plus slide-tape program accompanied by script. Payment required with order.

B174. UNIVERSITY OF ARIZONA—ARIZONA MEDICAL CENTER, Medical Audiovisual Services, Tucson, Ariz. 85724.*

PURPOSE. To produce audiovisual programs for instruction in health sciences. *Specialization:* audiovisual instruction in health sciences.
PUBLICATIONS. Among programs available are four slide-tape combinations on Down's syndrome, toxicology, postmaturity, and adolescent medicine—designed for medical students in clerkships and other interested medical and paramedical personnel. Payment not required with order.

B175. UNIVERSITY OF CALIFORNIA EXTENSION MEDIA CENTER, Berkeley, Calif. 94720. *Tel:* (415) 642-0460. C. Cameron Macauley, Dir.

PURPOSE. To rent and sell media for college and adult market. *Specialization:* instructional media.
PUBLICATIONS. Offerings described in pamphlets and newsletters of consistently outstanding graphical treatment. Extension Media Center's *Lifelong Learning* is magazine unto itself, describing currently available series of media offerings and presenting columns by experts in the fields in question. *Lifelong Learning* contains some of best written analyses of film and sound recording around, as well as articles on politics, women's studies, and academia. Hefty 300-page film catalog: capsule descriptions are actually mini-reviews, touching on films' weak as well as strong points. Dozens of titles in medical sciences for professional, medical student, and general audiences. Largest selections on treatment/healing/rehabilitation and diseases/pathology. Equally impressive selections in life sciences and psychology. Books, pamphlets, slides, records, and audio- and videotapes. Special brochure on health materials being prepared. Payment required with some orders.

UNIVERSITY OF CALIFORNIA—THE MEDICAL MEDIA NETWORK *See* B114

UNIVERSITY OF CHICAGO PRESS *See* G77

B176. UNIVERSITY OF CONNECTICUT, Center for Instructional Media and Technology, Storrs, Conn. 06268.* *Tel:* (203) 486-2530, 2531. Philip I. Sleeman, Dir.

PURPOSE. To rent educational films to groups and individuals. *Specialization:* 16mm educational films.
PUBLICATIONS. Catalog contains over 5,000 titles—most for school-age audiences.

B177. UNIVERSITY OF CONNECTICUT HEALTH CENTER, Biomedical Communications Department, Farmington, Conn. 06032* *Tel:* (203) 674-2433. Louis Audette, Dir.

PURPOSE. To offer a broad range of services in the preparation of audiovisual materials for instruction, publication, and research.
PUBLICATIONS. Produces media and a wide variety of graphics and illustration services to the Health Center, its affiliates, and outside clients. Manages interactive TV network. ˙

UNIVERSITY OF CONNECTICUT HEALTH CENTER *See* E41

B178. UNIVERSITY OF IOWA AUDIOVISUAL CENTER, Media Library, C-5 East Hall, Iowa City, Iowa 52240. *Tel:* (319) 353-5885. William Oglesby, Dir.

PURPOSE. To rent audiovisual materials. *Specialization:* audiovisual library.
SPECIAL INFORMATION SERVICES. *Languages:* French, Spanish, and German.
PUBLICATIONS. Hefty 500-page catalog with 1975 supplement. Films in health and hygiene, intended mostly for general audiences, cover nutrition, alcohol and drugs, venereal disease, posture, dental care, growth, and environment. Large selection in medicine in theories and principles, anatomy and physiology, pathology, microbiology, internal medicine, neurology, psychiatry, communicable disease, etc. Most medical films aimed at college and adult levels. Also good selection in dentistry. More advanced medical films deal with surgery and diagnosis, pharmaceuticals, health service administration, rehabilitation, and nursing. Separate price list (Section M). Section D price list covers dentistry—general, crown and bridge, prosthesis, oral surgery, etc. Also of interest is series of films on speech pathology, and modular concepts in human disease—basic instruction in package of tape cassettes and slides. Payment not required with order.

B179. UNIVERSITY OF MAINE FILM RENTAL LIBRARY, 16 Shibles Hall, Orono, Maine 04473. *Tel:* (207) 581-7541. John Henderson, Mgr.

PURPOSE. 16mm film resource center for the northeastern United States. *Specialization:* educational films.
SPECIAL INFORMATION SERVICE. *Special collection:* depository for Department of Health, Education, and Welfare titles.

PUBLICATIONS. Catalog put out every other year with supplements. Occasional pamphlets. Extensive variety and number of films on subjects from aeronautics to zoology. Health science subjects include animal diseases, plant and animal biology, first aid, nutrition, psychology, and microbiology. Free catalog gives good descriptions of several hundred films, along with recommended audience (primary grades through adult). Rental charge billed after film returned to library.

B180. UNIVERSITY OF MICHIGAN—AUDIO-VISUAL EDUCATION CENTER, 416 Fourth St., Ann Arbor, Mich. 48103. *Tel:* (313) 764-5360. Ford L. Lemler, Dir.

PURPOSE. To distribute educational materials on a low-cost rental basis for use by schools, institutions, community groups, etc. *Specialization:* educational films.
SPECIAL INFORMATION SERVICES. Information on films and/or sources of films in variety of curriculum areas.
PUBLICATIONS. Catalogs, indexes to catalogs, and supplements to catalogs of films, books, audiotapes, and filmstrips. Film catalog has several hundred titles; health and medical subjects are aimed at school-age audiences (biology, basic anatomy, hygiene). "From 'Abacus' to 'Zurich'" is an index to the descriptive catalog. Large and interesting selections of films. Payment not required with order.

UNIVERSITY OF NEBRASKA MEDICAL CENTER *See* B33

B181. UNIVERSITY OF NEW HAMPSHIRE—NEW ENGLAND HEALTH RESOURCES CENTER, Department of Media Services, Durham, N.H. 03824.* *Tel:* (603) 862-2240. John D. Bardwell, Media Services Dir.

PURPOSE. To provide audiovisual support to directors of hospital training and other health educators. *Specialization:* films on health for training.
PUBLICATIONS. Thirty-seven-page catalog of films available for rent from UNH. Many are aimed at general audiences. Payment not required with order.

B182. UNIVERSITY OF NORTH CAROLINA SCHOOL OF MEDICINE, Medical Television Center, Medical Sciences Teaching Laboratories, Chapel Hill, N.C. 27514.* David Raney, Dir., Medical TV Center.

PURPOSE. To produce audiovisual materials for the UNC Medical School. *Specialization:* audiovisual materials in health sciences.
PUBLICATIONS. Videotapes, audiotapes, films, and sound-slide sets in health sciences listed in large catalog are for use of UNC Medical School faculty, staff, and students.

B183. UNIVERSITY OF NORTH CAROLINA SCHOOL OF MEDICINE—SELF-INSTRUCTIONAL MATERIALS PROJECT, Trailer 16, Manning Dr., Chapel Hill, N.C. 27514.* *Tel:* (919) 966-2246, 2247. Rita B. Johnson, Project Ed.

PURPOSE. To produce multimedia packages for medical self-instruction. *Specialization:* self-instruction in medicine.
PUBLICATIONS. Packages are produced by consortium of southern medical colleges, which get 50 percent discount on packages. Newsletter (monthly) lists new packages. Payment not required with order.

B184. UNIVERSITY OF TEXAS—HEALTH SCIENCE CENTER AT SAN ANTONIO, Learning Resources Center, 7703 Floyd Curl Dr., San Antonio, Tex. 78284.* *Tel:* (512) 696-6271. Cynthia Robinson, Lib., Learning Resources Center.

PURPOSE. To maintain collection of health science audiovisuals for students and staff of the UT Health Science Center. *Specialization:* multimedia resources in health sciences.
PUBLICATIONS. 134-page index of holdings (audiocassettes, slide-sound programs, and films). Videotape catalog. For use of University of Texas medical professionals and students.

B185. UNIVERSITY OF WYOMING FILM LIBRARY, Box 3273 University Station, Laramie, Wyo. 82071.

PURPOSE. To distribute educational films. *Specialization:* educational films.
PUBLICATIONS. Supplements that can be used in conjunction with film catalog of Mountain Plains Educational Media Council. Supplements run about 35 pages; general health, hygiene, safety, and biology. Payment not required with order.

UPJOHN COMPANY *See* F34

WARD'S NATURAL SCIENCE ESTABLISHMENT, INC. *See* F35.

B186. WAYNE STATE UNIVERSITY, Systems, Distribution, and Utilization Department, 5448 Cass Ave., Detroit, Mich. 48202. *Tel:* (313) 577-1980.

PURPOSE. To distribute and produce audiovisual instructive materials. *Specialization:* audiovisual materials.
PUBLICATIONS. 350-page catalog of instructional materials, $2. Numerous films on medicine and health for both general and professional audiences. DENT Project (Directions in Education for Nursing via Technology) brings together kinescope films, videotapes, and study guides in 106 lessons on nursing skills: injections, bed-changing, nutrition, enemas, etc. Mimeographed supplements to catalog. Films are for rent. Payment not required with order.

B187. WEXLER FILM PRODUCTIONS, INC., 801 N. Seward St., Los Angeles, Calif. 90038. *Tel:* (213) 462-6671. Sy Wexler, Owner-Producer.

PURPOSE. To produce educational films with major interest in medicine and health. *Specialization:* medical films.
PUBLICATIONS. Films are aimed at professional audiences; 14-page catalog lists dozens of subjects—pharmacology, surgery, post-op, diagnosis, fractures, gynecology, lab apparatus, otology, etc. Payment not required with order.

WILEY BIOMEDICAL DIVISION *See* G88

WILLIAMS AND WILKINS COMPANY *See* G89

B188. XEROX EDUCATION PUBLICATIONS/XEROX FILMS, 245 Long Hill Rd., Middletown, Conn. 06457. *Tel:* (203) 347-7251. Gerald S. Isaacson, Pres.

PURPOSE. To develop and market printed and audiovisual products in the education community. *Specialization:* instructional books, films, and filmstrips.

PUBLICATIONS. Books, films, periodicals, and filmstrips. Well-illustrated and informative catalog with good descriptions of films and other materials with recommended audiences (elementary to adult). Films on animal and plant biology; filmstrip series on careers includes exploration of careers in health. Payment not required with order.

XEROX UNIVERSITY MICROFILMS *See* G91

YEAR BOOK MEDICAL PUBLISHERS *See* G92

C

Book Dealers

C1. ADLER'S FOREIGN BOOKS, 162 Fifth Ave., New York, N.Y. 10010. *Tel:* (212) 691-5151. George Thewman, Mgr.

PURPOSE. To distribute medical titles and magazines. *Specialization:* foreign-language books.
SPECIAL INFORMATION SERVICES. *Languages:* French, Spanish, German, Italian, Greek, and Latin.
PUBLICATIONS. Payment not required with order.

C2. BALLEN BOOKSELLERS INTERNATIONAL, INC., 66 Austin Blvd., Commack, N.Y. 11725. *Tel:* (516) 543-5600. Leonard Schrift, Pres.

PURPOSE. A bookseller to academic, medical, and research libraries. *Specialization:* books.
PUBLICATIONS. Offerings of dozens of publishing houses; seventy-page handbook on Ballen's Approval Plan for providing libraries with approval copies of all new publications in designated areas. Payment not required with order.

BARTEL DENTAL BOOK COMPANY *See* G13

C3. P. AND H. BLISS, Middletown, Conn. 06457. *Tel:* (203) 347-2255. Philip Bliss, Owner.

PURPOSE. To supply back issues of periodicals, journals, magazines, and serials.
PUBLICATIONS. Occasional catalog. Payment required with individual order.

C4. BOOKPEOPLE, 2940 Seventh St., Berkeley, Calif. 94701. *Tel:* (415) 549-3030. Richard Reiheld, Gen. Mgr.

PURPOSE. A wholesale distributor of trade and small-press books. *Specialization:* books.

PUBLICATIONS. Number of titles dealing with health aimed toward lay readers, with list of titles available on request. Little of interest to professionals.

C5. EBSCO SUBSCRIPTION SERVICES, Box 1943, Birmingham, Ala. 35201. *Tel:* (205) 252-1212. J. T. Stephens, Pres.

PURPOSE. To provide subscription service for serial publications from all nations. Deals with virtually any medical or related journal.

C6. ELIOT BOOKS, INC., 35-53 24 St., Long Island City, N.Y. 11951. *Tel:* (212) 937-2070. George Eliot, Pres.

PURPOSE. A book dealer meeting domestic book needs of health professionals, handling titles of the significant biomedical publishers. *Specialization:* books and serials on medicine.

PUBLICATIONS. Monthly newsletter with complete bibliographic information on all new books. Over 10,000 titles said to be in stock; orders will be filled in 24 hours, according to publicity. Four hundred and fifty series titles carried on clinical sciences, nursing science, pharmacy, veterinary science, and dentistry. Payment not required with order.

C7. W. BRUCE FYE, 307 Overbrook Rd., Baltimore, Md. 21212.*

PURPOSE. To sell old, rare, and out of print books with an emphasis on medical and scientific items.

PUBLICATIONS. Catalog has a subject index and is arranged by author. Most items are o.p. books at reasonable prices. Prepayment required except for libraries.

C8. WALTER J. JOHNSON, INC., 355 Chestnut St., Norwood, N.J. 07648. *Tel:* (201) 767-1303. Walter J. Johnson, Pres.

PURPOSE. To supply in-print books and back-issue periodicals to colleges, universities, and research libraries in all fields and subject areas in all languages. *Specialization:* reprints of books and periodicals.

PUBLICATIONS. Supplies originals of in-print titles, reprints of monographs and reference works, continuations, and second-hand rare and modern collections. Over 100,000 titles in periodicals, and will search for any serial back-set or run not in stock. Also single volumes and issues, reprints, and microforms. Central source reference supply service. Special subject bulletins and comprehensive catalogs. "English Experience" series reprints in facsimile books set in movable type in England, 1475–1640. Includes early books on anatomy and medicine. Payment required with order under $10.

C9. EMIL OFFENBACHER, OLD AND RARE BOOKS, 84-50 Austin St., Kew Gardens, N.Y. 11415. *Tel:* (212) 849-5834. Emil Offenbacher, Proprietor.

PURPOSE. An antiquarian bookseller. (Services restricted to rare book collectors and libraries.) *Specialization:* medicine and sciences.

SPECIAL INFORMATION SERVICES. *Special collections:* many pre-1840 medical and scientific volumes.
PUBLICATIONS. Catalogs of rare books (published once yearly). Payment required with orders from nonregular customers.

C10. OLD HICKORY BOOKSHOP, Brinklow, Md. 20727.* *Tel:* (301) 924-2225.

PURPOSE. To buy and sell old and rare medical books. A small dealer, Old Hickory has a fine reputation.
PUBLICATIONS. Produces lists of books available, arranged by author.

C11. JUNE O'SHEA BOOKS, 1206½ S. Roxbury Dr., Los Angeles, Calif. 90035. *Tel:* (213) 553-0678. June O'Shea, Owner.

PURPOSE. A bookseller of second-hand, out-of-print, or reprinted books and monographs. (Services restricted to universities, colleges, and criminal justice personnel.) *Specialization:* psychology and psychiatry.
PUBLICATIONS. Separate catalogs for psychology/psychiatry and criminology. Four thousand titles in former. Payment not required with order.

C12. ALBERT J. PHIEBIG, INC., Box 352, White Plains, N.Y. 10602. *Tel:* (914) WH 8-0138. Albert J. Phiebig, Pres.

PURPOSE. A bookseller to libraries.
PUBLICATIONS. Sells foreign books and periodicals, current and out of print. Irregular serials; international congresses' results. Payment required with subscription orders from institutions.

C13. RITTENHOUSE BOOK DISTRIBUTORS, INC., 251 S. 24 St., Philadelphia, Pa. 19103.*

PURPOSE. To distribute books from trade and university publishers, especially in medicine. *Specialization:* medical books.
PUBLICATIONS. Catalog of new titles available.

C14. HENRY SCHUMAN, LTD., 2211 Broadway, New York, N.Y. 10024. *Tel:* (212) SC 4-2393. Mrs. Henry Schuman, Pres.

PURPOSE. A dealer in rare books pertaining to the history of medicine and science. *Specialization:* history of medicine and science; many subjects in many periods.
SPECIAL INFORMATION SERVICES. *Languages:* English, French, Spanish, German, and Latin.
PUBLICATIONS. Three to four catalogs per year. Fascinating compendium of works from Aristotle to Max Planck, including many landmark works in medical science: first translations of Freud, Arab physicians, second edition of first book devoted to dentistry (*Zene Artzney*). Sold to private collectors or institutions. Payment required with order unless charge account established.

C15. YANKEE BOOK PEDDLER, Box 366, Fountain Sq., Contocook, N.H. 03229.* *Tel:* (603) 746-4090.

PURPOSE. "Devoted to the exclusive jobbing of all university presses to school, public and college libraries." *Specialization:* scholarly books.

PUBLICATIONS. *What's New in Scholarly Books*, a journal of reviews, is published quarterly. Covers medical books issued by university presses. Standing orders for entire output of one press, one series of the press, or by subject interest are accepted. Larger-than-normal discounts generally offered.

D

City, State, and Federal Agencies

D1. AEROMEDICAL RESEARCH LABORATORY LIBRARY, U.S. Army, Box 577, Fort Rucker, Ala. 36362. *Tel:* (205) 255-5109; AUTOVON 558-5109. Sybil H. Bullock, Librarian.

PURPOSE. To provide research and development materials in bioacoustics, aviation psychology, aviation medical research, biochemistry, engineering, and electronics. *Specialization:* aviation medical research, bioacoustics, aviation psychology, and safety.
SPECIAL INFORMATION SERVICES. *Special collections:* all Army Aeromedical Research Laboratory reports.
PUBLICATIONS. Technical reports in physiology, psychology, chemistry, engineering, safety, optics, and biomedical electronics as they pertain to aviation and flight. Also films, books, periodicals, pamphlets, and handbooks in these areas. Payment not required with order.

AIR POLLUTION TECHNICAL INFORMATION CENTER *See* E1

D2. AKRON CITY HEALTH DEPARTMENT, 177 S. Broadway, Akron, Ohio 44308. *Tel:* (216) 375-2960. Noble E. Sherrard, Interim Dir. of Health.

PURPOSE. To provide public health services, including immunization, health education, and environmental health programs. *Specialization:* public health.
SPECIAL INFORMATION SERVICES. Speakers, films, and health information for the public. *Special collections:* public health journals and books.
PUBLICATIONS. Pamphlets, slides, videotapes, periodicals. Payment not required with order.

D3. ARKANSAS DEPARTMENT OF HEALTH, 4815 W. Markham St., Little Rock, Ark. 72201. *Tel:* (501) 661-2000. Rex C. Ramsay, Dir.

PURPOSE. To promote and protect the health of the citizens of Arkansas. (Services restricted to citizens of Arkansas.) *Specialization:* public health and safety.
PUBLICATIONS. Illustrated report on activities and disbursements; department services brochure; 80-page film catalog—free rental films for groups and individuals, dozens of titles on health, safety, growing up, and communicable diseases. Also filmstrips.
INQUIRY ADDRESS. Mrs. Daisye Zimmerman, Dir., Div. of Public Health Education, 4815 W. Markham St., Little Rock, Ark. 72201. *Tel:* (501) 661-2351.

D4. ARMED FORCES INSTITUTE OF PATHOLOGY—DEPARTMENT OF THE ARMY, Washington, D.C. 20306. Col. James L. Hansen, M.D., Dir.

PURPOSE. To publish instructional materials in pathology as it relates to armed forces medicine. *Specialization:* pathology.
SPECIAL INFORMATION SERVICES. Consultation service. Pathologic material loaned to institutions and medical professionals. Medical illustrative material. Note: services are not restricted to armed forces health personnel. Institute serves both government and civilian organizations.
PUBLICATIONS. *Commanders Digest* (periodical). List of educational aids runs to 144 pages and lists microscope slides, lantern slides, cases, and films. Many films for military use only. *Atlas of Tumor Pathology,* syllabi, manuals, and textbooks. Special publication on Billings Collection of antique microscopes in Armed Forces Medical Museum. Payment required with order.

D5. BALTIMORE CITY HEALTH DEPARTMENT, Room 201-A, Health Information, 111 N. Calvert St., Baltimore, Md. 21202. John B. De Hoff, Commissioner.

PURPOSE. A public health department with the duties of inspection and information. *Specialization:* public health.
PUBLICATIONS. Extensive range of materials. Everything from measles to toothaches are dealt with in publications. Extensive information on controlling rats. Child care, venereal disease, communicable diseases, hygiene, drugs, and all areas of health explained for general public in pamphlets, folders, charts, stick-on labels, and flyers. Much of local interest for Baltimore area residents, but general information also provided. Most materials free.

D6. BUREAU OF HEALTH MANPOWER, U.S. Department of Health, Education, and Welfare, 9000 Rockville Pike, Bethesda, Md. 20014. *Tel:* (301) 496-6011. Daniel Whiteside, D.D.S., Dir. Bureau of Health Manpower.

PURPOSE. To coordinate, evaluate, and support development and utilization of nation's health workers. *Specialization:* health manpower.
PUBLICATIONS. Twelve-page publications list of booklets, books, films, and slides concentrating on careers in health, manpower needs, guides to further films and books, statistics, medicine, nursing, dentistry, and allied health professions. Single copies free.

D7. CENTER FOR DISEASE CONTROL, U.S. Department of Health, Education, and Welfare, Public Health Service, Atlanta, Ga. 30333.

PURPOSE. A federal agency for research, information, and coordination with other institutions on infectious diseases, their causes and transmittal. *Specialization:* infectious diseases.

SPECIAL INFORMATION SERVICES. Wide range of services for general public and other health institutions and government agencies. Statistical reports, recommendation of standards, surveys, diagnoses, consultation in United States and abroad, physical examinations, training health-care workers, and more.

PUBLICATIONS. Free pamphlets on role of center. Individual pamphlets on diseases— hepatitis, influenza, mumps, venereal disease, rubella, rabies, tetanus, meningococcal meningitis, ringworm, malaria, and disease-transmitting insects. Center also involved in research on lesser known diseases that affect mainly persons in foreign countries, especially West African nations. Most materials free (single copies).

D8. DEFENSE CIVIL PREPAREDNESS AGENCY, Pentagon, Washington, D.C. 20301. *Tel:* (202) OX 5-9442. John E. Davis, Dir.

PURPOSE. To provide jointly with states for a civil defense system for protection of property and life in the United States in the event of nuclear attack. Also publishes information on coping with natural disasters. *Specialization:* civil defense.

PUBLICATIONS. Manuals on protecting oneself in event of attack by enemy nations. Materials cover fallout shelters, emergency medical care, sanitation, survival. Also information on survival in storms, tornadoes, earthquakes, and other disasters. Bimonthly magazine *Foresight*, with articles on similar topics and new developments. Sixty-five-page catalog of publications—handbooks, abstracts, and pamphlets. Motion picture catalog with several dozen films for free loan or for purchase; these are public information films as opposed to training aids (available separately) and cover mainly natural disasters. Also slides and radio-TV spots. Most materials free.

INQUIRY ADDRESS. Information Services, DCPA, Pentagon, Washington, D.C. 20301. *Tel:* (202) OX 5-9442.

D9. FEDERAL AVIATION ADMINISTRATION, Department of Transportation, Washington, D.C. 20591.*

PURPOSE. A federal regulatory agency for insuring safety in air travel and transport. *Specialization:* aviation safety.

PUBLICATIONS. 16mm films, sound-slide programs, and filmstrips (including some on safety) available for purchase or free loan. Catalog.

D10. FOOD AND DRUG ADMINISTRATION, Consumer Inquiries, HFG-20, 5600 Fisher Lane, Rockville, Md. 20852. *Tel:* (301) 443-3170. Ruth Beeler White, Dir., Consumer Inquiries.

PURPOSE. The Department of Health, Education, and Welfare's consumer protection agency. *Specialization:* consumer affairs.

PUBLICATIONS. *FDA Consumer*, ten issues per year (official magazine of FDA); *Consumer Memos* list brochures on fair labeling, packaging, food additives, food poisoning, drugs, and medicines; index of selected federal publications on similar topics, available from Public Documents Distribution Center. Also films. Payment required only with order for *FDA Consumer.*

D11. HAWAII STATE DEPARTMENT OF HEALTH, Health Education Office, Box 3378, Honolulu, Hawaii 96801. *Tel:* (808) 548-5886. Christine Ling, Health Education Officer.

PURPOSE. A state public health agency. (Services restricted to Hawaiians.)
PUBLICATIONS. Pamphlets; *Hawaii Health Messenger* (quarterly), newsletter of state interest. Illustrated annual report.

D12. LIBRARY OF CONGRESS, Catalog Publication Division, Washington, D.C. 20540.* William J. Welsh, Dir., Processing Dept.

PURPOSE. To issue guides to holdings in the Library of Congress's audiovisual collection and to materials available elsewhere. *Specialization:* catalogs of films and other projected materials.
PUBLICATIONS. Guide to availability of *Films and Other Materials for Projection* runs 175 pages, with hundreds of titles. User must order from sources indicated in catalog, not from LC, but LC will send catalog cards or MARC tapes. Large selection of offerings in health (mostly hygiene) and anatomy. For $40/yr., subscriber receives three quarterly film catalogs and annual cumulation. Payment required with order.

D13. LIBRARY OF CONGRESS DIVISION FOR THE BLIND AND PHYSICALLY HANDICAPPED, 1291 Taylor St. N.W., Washington, D.C. 20542. *Tel:* (202) 882-5500. Frank Kurt Cylke, Div. Chief.

PURPOSE. To provide free library service of books and magazines in recorded and braille formats for persons unable to read standard print materials because of visual or physical impairment. (Services restricted to residents of the United States and American citizens living abroad who are unable to read regular-print materials through visual impairment.) *Specialization:* braille and recorded publications.
SPECIAL INFORMATION SERVICES. Answers questions on various aspects of blindness and physical handicaps (except strictly medical and legal matters).
PUBLICATIONS. Cumulated catalogs and bimonthly magazines *Talking Book Topics*, *Braille Book Review*, and *New Braille Musician*. Lists of new materials recently added to collection. Medical and health topics are aimed at nonprofessional readers.

D14. NATIONAL AGRICULTURAL LIBRARY—U.S. DEPARTMENT OF AGRICULTURE, 10301 Baltimore Blvd., Beltsville, Md. 20705. *Tel:* (301) 344-3719. Richard A. Farley, Dir.

PURPOSE. To serve the research needs of Department of Agriculture personnel and others with interest in library's resources. *Specialization:* agriculture and nutrition.
SPECIAL INFORMATION SERVICES. CAIN-On-Line computer-search bibliographies. Customized bibliographies and referral services for FNIC users.
PUBLICATIONS. Food and Nutrition Information and Educational Materials Center has collection of materials useful in training personnel in food management for schools and other programs. Material provided on loan to school and other food service personnel includes films, videocassettes, audiotapes, pamphlets, books and reprints. FNIC users have access to total resources of National Agricultural Library. Most services free.

D15. NATIONAL AUDIOVISUAL CENTER, GENERAL SERVICES ADMIN-ISTRATION, Washington, D.C. 20409. *Tel:* (301) 763-7420. Arthur F. Sampson, Admin.

PURPOSE. A division of the National Archives and Records Service, charged with producing and distributing audiovisual materials. *Specialization:* audiovisual educational material.
SPECIAL INFORMATION SERVICES. *Languages:* English and Spanish.
PUBLICATIONS. Impressive 350-page catalog of U.S government-produced audiovisuals. Hundreds of films and filmstrips in medicine alone—diagnosis, surgery, careers in medicine, military medicine, veterinary medicine, dentistry, microbiology. Most are for professional or medical student audiences; materials for general audiences listed under health and safety. Biology, psychology, and other related titles fill many pages. Separate catalog of 16mm color films from Atomic Energy Commission includes radiology and animal life. Health, Education, and Welfare Department films also covered in information from GSA. National Medical Audiovisual Center newsletter details newly available films; of interest are teaching units using slides and audiotapes and slide/sound programs explaining MEDLARS and MEDLINE. Materials for purchase and rent. Payment required with order.

D16. NATIONAL CENTER FOR HEALTH STATISTICS, U.S. Public Health Service, 5600 Fishers Lane, Rockville, Md. 20852. *Tel:* (301) 443-1200. Edward B. Perrin, Dir.

PURPOSE. A part of U.S. Public Health Service's Health Resources Administration. *Specialization:* health statistics.
PUBLICATIONS. Report on center's activities; supplements to main catalog of publications; notes on new publications; current listing and topical index to "Vital and Health Statistics" series. Statistics cover mortality, expenses, facilities, and provide complete profile in numbers of health systems in the United States. Also data tapes. Single copies free, data tapes sold.
INQUIRY ADDRESS. Scientific and Technical Information Branch, National Center for Health Statistics, U.S. Public Health Service, 5600 Fishers Lane, Rockville, Md. 20852. *Tel:* (301) 443-1200.

D17. NATIONAL INSTITUTE OF CHILD HEALTH AND HUMAN DEVEL-OPMENT, U.S. Department of Health, Education, and Welfare, Bethesda, Md. 20014. Gerald D. LaVeck, Dir.

PURPOSE. A government agency, part of the National Institutes of Health, promoting research and making available information on growth, health, learning, and welfare of children, and on such topics as aging. *Specialization:* child health and human development.
SPECIAL INFORMATION SERVICES. *Languages:* English and Spanish.
PUBLICATIONS. Attractive booklets for general readers explain menopause and aging and their relationship to incidence of mongolism in newborn children and their effects on bodily well-being. Also booklet on sudden infant death syndrome (proceedings of conference) and illustrated report on ongoing research supported by the Institute of Child Health. NIH publications list of 48 pages with offerings of all

institutes under NIH umbrella: cancer, eye, heart and lung, dental institutes, National Library of Medicine, etc. Single copies generally free from issuing institute or office, otherwise can be purchased from Superintendent of Documents.

D18. NATIONAL INSTITUTE OF DENTAL RESEARCH, National Institutes of Health, Bethesda, Md. 20014. *Tel:* (301) 496-4261. Tula S. Brocard, Chief Executive Officer.

PURPOSE. A federal research institution sponsoring basic lab and clinical research into causes and prevention of oral-facial diseases and disorders. *Specialization:* dental research.

PUBLICATIONS. "Research Explores . . ." series of pamphlets on nutrition and dental health, dental decay, pyorrhea, plaque, canker sores and fever blisters, cleft palate, and tooth care. Pamphlets are illustrated and clearly written for general readership. Single copies free. Payment required with bulk orders, which go to Government Printing Office.

D19. NATIONAL INSTITUTES OF HEALTH, 9000 Rockville Pike, Bethesda, Md. 20014. *Tel:* (301) 656-4000. Donald S. Frederickson, M.D., Dir.

PURPOSE. Under the Department of Health, Education, and Welfare, a government agency conducting and supporting biomedical research. *Specialization:* medical research.

SPECIAL INFORMATION SERVICES. News releases, announcements prepared for general press and scientific media; publications prepared for general public and scientific community.

PUBLICATIONS. Informational pamphlet on functions of NIH; 50-page publications list; *1975 Almanac* with statistics and chronology of government action in field of health since 1783; *Research Advancements* is large-format 100-page, professionally produced round-up of events and breakthroughs in current medical scene. NIH produces comprehensive and complete studies in all areas of medical research. Medical professionals will find almost anything they need in NIH publications. Payment not required with order. Single free copies available in most instances, bulk copies purchased from Government Printing Office.

INQUIRY ADDRESS. Division of Public Information, National Institutes of Health, 9000 Rockville Pike, Bethesda, Md. 20014. *Tel:* (301) 496-5787.

D20. NATIONAL LIBRARY OF MEDICINE, 8600 Rockville Pike, Bethesda, Md. 20014.* *Tel:* (301) 656-4000.

PURPOSE. "To assist in the advancement of medical and related sciences by the collection, dissemination, and exchange of scientific and other information important to the progress of medicine and public health."

SPECIAL INFORMATION SERVICES. Interlibrary loans through the Biomedical Communications Network and other libraries; the National Medical Audiovisual Center (see D21); and an extramural program that administers grant support. *Special collections:* numerous special collections include an incunabula collection of over 500 volumes.

PUBLICATIONS. Numerous indexes generated from the MEDLARS (medical literature analysis and retrieval system) which began in 1964. Most notable are *Index Medicus, Index to Dental Literature,* and *International Nursing Index.*

D21. NATIONAL MEDICAL AUDIOVISUAL CENTER, Public Health Service, Department of Health, Education, and Welfare, 1600 Clifton Rd., Atlanta, Ga. 30333. *Tel:* (404) 633-3351. George E. Mitchell, D.M.D., Dir.

PURPOSE. To conduct programs in media development, acquisition, consultation, training, and educational research, and to provide short-term film loans for educational use. *Specialization:* films for medical instruction.
PUBLICATIONS. 180-page film catalog can be purchased only from Superintendent of Documents, Washington, D.C. ($3.05 in U.S.) Several hundred films for use in professional educational programs in the health sciences. Largest selections in clinical pathology, dentistry, and paraplegia; nursing and rehabilitation also covered. Films from government agencies, medical schools, and clinics. Films on history of medicine might appeal to general audiences. Payment not required with order.

D22. NEW YORK STATE HEALTH DEPARTMENT, Tower Building, Empire State Plaza, Albany, N.Y. 12237. *Tel:* (518) 474-2029. Robert P. Whalen, M.D., Commissioner.

PURPOSE. A state agency for protecting the health of New York State residents and visitors. *Specialization:* public health.
PUBLICATIONS. Publications catalog with 14 pages listing printed material. Pamphlets for general audiences on health and hygiene; others for health professionals, mostly in areas of public health and administration. Posters and charts can be ordered. Other catalogs on exhibits, films, and professional films. Single copies of materials free to New York State residents. Payment not required with bulk order.
INQUIRY ADDRESS. Office of Health Communications and Education, New York State Health Department, Tower Building, Empire State Plaza, Albany, N.Y. 12237. *Tel:* (518) 474-2029.

D23. OHIO RIVER VALLEY WATER SANITATION COMMISSION (ORSANCO), 414 Walnut St., Cincinnati, Ohio 45202. *Tel:* (513) 421-1151. Leo Weaver, Exec. Dir.

PURPOSE. An interjurisdictional government agency to abate water pollution in Ohio River Basin. *Specialization:* water pollution abatement.
MEMBERSHIP. *Requirements:* commission appointed by heads of eight member states.
PUBLICATIONS. Annotated bibliography lists publications and special reports related to commission investigations; information on biological effects of water pollution, including fish kills, reports from Aquatic-Life Advisory Committee. *Quality Monitor* (monthly); annual reports also published. Payment required with order.

D24. THE PRESIDENT'S COMMITTEE ON EMPLOYMENT OF THE HANDICAPPED, Washington, D.C. 20210. *Tel:* (202) 961-3401. Harold Russell, Chmn.

PURPOSE. A government agency for information and education on employment for handicapped persons. *Specialization:* employment information regarding the handicapped.

PUBLICATIONS. Wide range of pamphlets and booklets concentrating on building design for the handicapped, guides for local and state committees in planning media campaigns, bibliography of guidebooks for handicapped travelers here and abroad, employment assistance for businesses, advice for the handicapped applying for jobs. *Opening Doors for the Handicapped* lists films and three-dimensional exhibits available from state and federal sources. Committee is source for ad copy and radio spot announcements also. Payment usually not required with order.

D25. REHABILITATION SERVICES ADMINISTRATION, Social and Rehabilitation Service, U.S. Department of Health, Education, and Welfare, Washington, D.C. 20201.

PURPOSE. To support state-federal program of rehabilitation programs and special grants relating to mental retardation and other developmental disabilities. *Specialization:* rehabilitation.

PUBLICATIONS. Thirty-two-page directory of SRS publications. Information on community services, assistance for the poor, statistics, manpower studies, volunteer work, Medicaid, and all aspects of rehabilitation for the blind, retarded, disabled, and aged. Some single copies free; others purchased from Government Printing Office.

D26. SOCIAL AND ECONOMIC STATISTICS ADMINISTRATION, Bureau of the Census, U.S Department of Commerce, Washington, D.C. 20233. Vincent P. Barabba, Dir.

PURPOSE. A government agency for the compilation of statistics on nation's industrial production and trade and on population. *Specialization:* population and commerce.

PUBLICATIONS. Yearly catalogs of various reports, abstracts, charts, and profiles, plus cumulative catalog of reports since first national census in 1790. Concentration on trade, including manufacture of pharmaceuticals, medical instruments, and supplies. Demographic publications outline birth and death rates, in-migration, immigration, racial makeup of nation, and other facts. Payment required with order; order from Superintendent of Documents, Washington, D.C. 20402.

D27. STATE OF CALIFORNIA DEPARTMENT OF HEALTH, 744 P St., Sacramento, Calif. 95814.*

PURPOSE. A California state health agency offering free-loan films to groups in state. *Specialization:* films on health.

PUBLICATIONS. Sixty-five-page catalog of 16mm films, sound and silent filmstrips, and slides.

D28. STATE OF MAINE DEPARTMENT OF HEALTH AND WELFARE, State House, Augusta, Maine 04333. *Tel:* (207) 289-3707. David Smith, Commissioner.

PURPOSE. To provide information and education services for the department. *Specialization:* public relations in field of health.

PUBLICATIONS. Pamphlets, films, slides, records, videotapes, and periodicals.

INQUIRY ADDRESS. Katy Perry, State of Maine Department of Health and Welfare, State House, Augusta, Maine 04333. *Tel:* (207) 289-3707.

E

Libraries and Information Services

AEROMEDICAL RESEARCH LABORATORY LIBRARY *See* D1

E1. AIR POLLUTION TECHNICAL INFORMATION CENTER, Environmental Protection Agency, Research Triangle Park, N.C. 27711. *Tel:* (919) 549-8411. Peter Halpin, Chief.

PURPOSE. To collect and disseminate information on air pollution, its effects, and prevention and control as reported in the literature. *Specialization:* air pollution.
SPECIAL INFORMATION SERVICES. Computerized literature searching, referrals, etc.
PUBLICATIONS. Periodicals. Payment required with order; order from Government Printing Office.

AKRON CITY HEALTH DEPARTMENT *See* D2

E2. THE ALBANY MEDICAL COLLEGE—UNION UNIVERSITY, Schaffer Library of Health Sciences, New Scotland Ave., Albany, N.Y. 12208. *Tel:* (518) 445-5530. Mrs. Ursula Poland, Librarian.

PURPOSE. To provide information services for the affiliates of the Medical College and Hospital. (Services open to outsiders for reference only.)
SPECIAL INFORMATION SERVICES. Computerized bibliographies. *Special collections:* medicine, preclinical science, and nursing.

E3. ALBERT EINSTEIN COLLEGE OF MEDICINE, D. Samuel Gottesman Library, Yeshiva University, 1300 Morris Park Ave., Bronx, N.Y. 10461.

PURPOSE. To serve research and teaching needs of students, faculty, and staff, as well as physicians and scientists of neighboring communities. *Specialization:* medicine and science.

115

SPECIAL INFORMATION SERVICES. *Special collections:* history of medicine and rare books.
PUBLICATIONS. Lists of new acquisitions and journals.

ALEXANDER GRAHAM BELL ASSOCIATION *See* A7

AMERICAN ASSOCIATION OF ORTHODONTISTS *See* A31

AMERICAN FOUNDATION FOR THE BLIND *See* A51

AMERICAN LIBRARY ASSOCIATION *See* A58

AMERICAN MEDICAL RECORD ASSOCIATION *See* A61

ARKANSAS DEPARTMENT OF HEALTH *See* D3

ARMED FORCES INSTITUTE OF PATHOLOGY *See* D4

E4. AUBURN UNIVERSITY LIBRARY, Auburn, Ala. 36830. *Tel:* (205) 826-4500. William C. Highfill, Dir.

PURPOSE. To serve university students and researchers.
SPECIAL INFORMATION SERVICES. MEDLINE computer search, Chemical and Biological Abstracts.

BALTIMORE CITY HEALTH DEPARTMENT *See* D5.

E5. BRAIN INFORMATION SERVICE, Center for the Health Sciences, University of California, Los Angeles, Calif. 90024. *Tel:* (213) 825-6011. Michael H. Chase, Dir.

PURPOSE. A part of the Neurological Information Network of the National Institute of Neurological Diseases and Stroke. Under the auspices of UCLA School of Medicine, BIS centrally catalogs the enormous volume of neuroscientific literature produced around the world and provides professional information analyses to researchers. *Specialization:* neurological sciences.
SPECIAL INFORMATION SERVICES. Customized bibliographies.
PUBLICATIONS. Annual announcements describe materials and activities of BIS. Service is involved with neurochemistry, -endocrinology -pharmacology, -anatomy, -physiology, sleep, and behavior. Provides individualized custom bibliographies drawn from computer file of 300,000 citations covering 1969 to the present for $25 fee. Conference reports, annual bibliographic volumes, *Sleep Bulletin* with reviews and bibliographies, results of symposia. Payment required with order.

BUREAU OF HEALTH MANPOWER *See* D6

E6. BUTLER UNIVERSITY, BUTLER SCIENCE LIBRARY, Indianapolis, Ind. 46208. *Tel:* (317) 283-9401. Miss C. Leibenguth, Science Librarian.

PURPOSE. To serve the students and faculty of the science departments of Butler University. (Services restricted to Butler faculty, staff, and students.)

SPECIAL INFORMATION SERVICES. *Special collections:* pharmacy collection and drug abuse materials.

CENTER FOR DISEASE CONTROL *See* D7

E7. CHEMICAL ABSTRACTS SERVICE, Division of American Chemical Society, Ohio State University, Columbus, Ohio 43210. *Tel:* (614) 421-6940. Dale B. Baker, Chief Executive Officer.

PURPOSE. To provide access to world's literature in chemistry and chemical engineering. *Specialization:* chemistry and chemical engineering.
PUBLICATIONS. Computer-readable data files which cover energy, materials, food and agricultural chemistry, ecology and environment; *Chemical Abstracts.* Brochures describe information services and fees. Payment required with order.
INQUIRY ADDRESS. Marketing Department, Chemical Abstracts Service, Ohio State University, Columbus, Ohio 43210. *Tel:* (614) 421-6940.

E8. CHICAGO COLLEGE OF OSTEOPATHIC MEDICINE—MEDICAL LIBRARY, 5200 Ellis Ave., Chicago, Ill. 60615. *Tel:* (312) 363-6800, ext. 487. Lee Brooke, Dir. of Libraries.

PURPOSE. Existing library collects audiotape cassettes and color slides as well as print materials. Library scheduled to open in January 1977 will be multimedia learning center for medical and paramedical students, staff, and faculty. *Specialization:* medicine and osteopathic medicine.
SPECIAL INFORMATION Services. *Special collections:* 1,500 cassette audiotapes (mostly Audio Digest); 1,500 color slides (mostly MEDCOM).

E9. COLORADO STATE UNIVERSITY LIBRARIES, Fort Collins, Colo. 80523. *Tel:* (303) 491-5911. Dr. L. W. Anderson, Dir.

PURPOSE. To support education, research, and service activities of Colorado State University.
SPECIAL INFORMATION SERVICES. *Special collections:* veterinary medicine.

E10. CORNELL UNIVERSITY MEDICAL COLLEGE LIBRARY, 1300 York Ave., New York, N.Y. 10021. *Tel:* (212) 472-6003. Erich Meyerhoff, Dir.

PURPOSE. To service students and staff of New York Hospital–Cornell Medical Center. (Services restricted to staff and students of New York Hospital–Cornell Medical Center and affiliated institutions.)
SPECIAL INFORMATION SERVICES. State University of New York Biomedical Communication Network and MEDLINE (National Library of Medicine), both computerized information services. *Special collections:* Medical archives has historical record of practice of medicine in the United States.

COUNCIL OF PLANNING LIBRARIANS EXCHANGE BIBLIOGRAPHIES *See* A118

E11. CREIGHTON UNIVERSITY—HEALTH SCIENCES LIBRARY, Learning Resources Center, Omaha, Nebr. 68131.* *Tel:* (402) 536-2908.

PURPOSE. To maintain audiovisual collection in health for use of Creighton faculty, staff, and students. *Specialization:* audiovisual collection in health sciences.
PUBLICATIONS. Forty-page list of programs. Videotapes, slides, and films.

E12. DARTMOUTH COLLEGE—DANA BIOMEDICAL LIBRARY, Hanover, N.H. 03755. *Tel:* (603) 646-2858. Shirley J. Grainger, Biomedical Librarian.

PURPOSE. To serve the students, faculty, and staff of Dartmouth College and Dartmouth-Hitchcock Medical Center (Dartmouth Medical School, Mary Hitchcock Memorial Hospital, Hitchcock Clinic, and White River Junction, Vt., VA Hospital). Serves the health sciences community of New Hampshire also. (Reference services and computer services restricted to New Hampshire and Vermont, apart from enquiries related to history of Dartmouth College and Medical School.) $100/yr. for guest-borrower card that enables non-Dartmouth community to borrow materials directly.
SPECIAL INFORMATION SERVICES. MEDLINE; access through NASIC to such data bases as Psychological Abstracts, CAIN, CHEMCON. *Special collections:* Raymond Pearl Collection on Longevity; Conner Collection of Rare Medical Classics; large collection of pre-1870 books.

E13. DEPARTMENT OF ARTIFICIAL ORGANS, Cleveland Clinic, 9500 Euclid Ave., Cleveland, Ohio 44106. *Tel:* (216) 229-2200. Yukihiko Nosé, Department Head.

PURPOSE. A hospital department for assembling and supplying information related to artificial organs, such as dialyzer, oxygenator, and circulatory assistance device. *Specialization:* artificial organs.

DRUG ABUSE COUNCIL *See* A120

E14. ENVIRONMENT INFORMATION CENTER, INC., 124 E. 39 St., New York, N.Y. 10016.*

PURPOSE. "An independent research and publishing organization that provides comprehensive intelligence, reporting, reference, and retrieval services covering all aspects of environmental affairs."
SPECIAL INFORMATION SERVICES. Will perform demand searches.
PUBLICATIONS. *Environment Abstracts* ($175/yr.), *Environment Index* ($75), *Environment Film Review* ($20), handbooks, microfiche of documents, and computer tape services. All cover health aspects of environment.

FELS RESEARCH INSTITUTE *See* H4.

E15. FIND/SVP HEALTHCARE INFORMATION CENTER, 500 Fifth Ave., New York, N.Y. 10036.* *Tel:* (212) 354-2424. Haines B. Gaffner, Pres.

PURPOSE. A "one-source information clearinghouse" on health matters for health-care industries and health professionals. *Specialization:* information searches in health.

SPECIAL INFORMATION SERVICES. Answers to inquiries in health culled from international sources.
PUBLICATIONS. Brochure describing subscription setup, which is available to executives and other professionals. Center engages in custom information searches on such questions as effects of chemicals on metabolism, status of health legislation, use of particular electronic devices, manufacturers of particular drugs or instruments, and similar inquiries. Calls handled confidentially. Monthly fees range $70–$300. Fees for projects can be quoted in advance if research is not covered by monthly subscription fee. Monthly newsletter *FINDOUT* sent to subscribers to services. Payment not required with subscription order.

E16. HARVARD UNIVERSITY, Francis A. Countway Library of Medicine (Boston Medical Library and Harvard Medical Library), 10 Shattuck St., Boston, Mass. 02115.* *Tel:* (617) 734-8900.

PURPOSE. To serve the Schools of Medicine, Public Health, and Dentistry of Harvard University and members of the Boston Medical Library. Also serves as New England Regional Medical Library Service.
SPECIAL INFORMATION SERVICES. *Special Collections:* general collection together with special collections numbers 450,000 plus volumes. Special collections in Chinese and Japanese medicine, Americana, and others.

E17. HEALTH INSURANCE INSTITUTE, 277 Park Ave., New York, N.Y. 10017. *Tel:* (212) 922-3000. Jim Williams, Chief Executive Officer.

PURPOSE. To serve as central source of health insurance information for the public. *Specialization:* health insurance plans, mortality and morbidity.
PUBLICATIONS. Pamphlets on trends, costs, and statistics in nation's health insurance industry; actuarial data. Single copies free.
INQUIRY ADDRESS. Library, Health Insurance Institute, 277 Park Ave., New York, N.Y. 10017. *Tel:* (212) 922-3022, 3024.

E18. HOWARD UNIVERSITY—MEDICAL-DENTAL LIBRARY, Health Sciences Center, Washington, D.C. 20059. *Tel:* (202) 636-6433.

PURPOSE. To serve the Health Sciences Center of Howard University, which includes teaching-hospital. (Services restricted to personnel at Howard University Health Sciences Center and to other health sciences libraries.) *Specialization:* basic and clinical sciences in medicine, dentistry, nursing, pharmacy, and allied health.
SPECIAL INFORMATION SERVICES. *Special collections:* the Negro in medicine and allied sciences.
PUBLICATIONS. Lists of available audiovisual materials in medicine and dentistry. Pamphlets, films, slides, audio- and videotapes, microforms, and transparencies.

E19. IDAHO STATE UNIVERSITY LIBRARY, Pocatello, Idaho 83209. *Tel:* (208) 236-3480. Eli M. Oboler, University Librarian.

PURPOSE. To provide library services to faculty and students of Idaho State for their curricular and research needs.

SPECIAL INFORMATION SERVICES. *Special Collections:* pharmacy, dental hygiene, speech pathology and audiology, nursing, radiological technology, and health-care administration.
INQUIRY ADDRESS. Interlibrary Loan Clerk, ISU Library, Pocatello, Idaho 83209. *Tel:* (208) 236-2494.

E20. ILLINOIS STATE UNIVERSITY—MILNER LIBRARY, Normal, Ill. 61761. *Tel:* (309) 436-8302.

PURPOSE. To support undergraduate and graduate programs at Illinois State University. (Services primarily for use by faculty, students, and administration of the university.) *Specialization:* university library, with some health materials.
SPECIAL INFORMATION SERVICES. *Special collections:* approximately 6,000 post-1967 volumes, 200 current periodicals, 50 current annuals, focusing on general field of medicine.
PUBLICATIONS. Descriptive brochures on use of library and on library's collections. *Periodicals Directory. ISU Theses Directory, Books in Storage.* Materials for in-house use only.
INQUIRY ADDRESS. Reference Department, Milner Library, Illinois State University, Normal, Ill. 61761. *Tel:* (309) 438-2204.

E21. INFORMATION CENTER FOR HEARING, SPEECH, AND DISORDERS OF HUMAN COMMUNICATION, B-2 Wood Basic Science Building, The Johns Hopkins Medical Institutions, Baltimore, Md. 21205. *Tel:* (301) 955-3390. Lois F. Lunin and Michael S. Weiss, Ph.D., Co-dirs.

PURPOSE. To serve as a national focal point for the identification, collection, storage, retrieval, analysis, repackaging, and dissemination of information on hearing, language, speech, and human communication, including reading disabilities. *Specialization:* alerting bulletins, bibliographies, and books on hearing, speech, and communications disorders.
SPECIAL INFORMATION SERVICES. Customized data base searches.
PUBLICATIONS. Two awareness services (Hearing and Balance; Language, Speech, and Voice) provide bulletins containing citations from journals, monographs, reports, which user can then go ahead and consult. Current issues available for libraries, back issues can be ordered. (New subscriptions not being accepted.) Biblio-Profiles provide concise state-of-the-art reports and bibliographies of recent articles. Conventional bibliographies, as well as monographs and special publications, are also carried. Information on where to obtain proceedings of workshops provided. Cumulated citations on hearing, speech, and communication disorders have been compiled for 1973 and 1974. Most publications can be ordered directly from Information Center. Payment required with order.
INQUIRY ADDRESS. Doc Sales, B-2 Wood Basic Science Building, The Johns Hopkins Medical Institutions, Baltimore, Md. 21205.

E22. INTERNATIONAL LIBRARY, ARCHIVES AND MUSEUM OF OPTOMETRY, 7000 Chippewa St., St. Louis, Mo. 63119 *Tel:* (314) 832-5558. Maria Dablemont, Librarian/Archivist.

PURPOSE. To provide optometric information and documentation with full library services. (Archival services restricted to qualified researchers.)
SPECIAL INFORMATION SERVICES. *Special collections:* vision science and related disciplines, with emphasis on optometry.

E23. JOHNS HOPKINS UNIVERSITY, WILLIAM H. WELCH MEDICAL LIBRARY, 1900 E. Monument St., Baltimore, Md. 21205. *Tel:* (301) 955-3411. Dr. Richard A. Polacsek, Dir./Librarian.

PURPOSE. A central resource library for the Johns Hopkins medical institutions. (Services restricted to Hopkins personnel.)
SPECIAL INFORMATION SERVICES. Multi-Media Learning Center; MEDLARS (National Library of Medicine); State University of New York Biomedical Communications Network.

E24. KANSAS STATE UNIVERSITY—VETERINARY MEDICAL LIBRARY, Kansas State University, Manhattan, Kans. 66506. *Tel:* (913) 532-5673. Guy Coffee, Veterinary Medical Librarian.

PURPOSE. To serve the needs of faculty, staff, and students of the College of Veterinary Medicine. (Services are nonrestricted except for borrowing privileges of audiovisual materials.) *Specialization:* veterinary and comparative medicine. Also contains basic core collection in basic and preclinical sciences.
SPECIAL INFORMATION SERVICES. Slide-tape presentations and audiotape cassettes. Book collections of over 11,000 volumes, 650 serial titles. *Special collections:* approximately two-fifths of collection is oriented to biomedical sciences.
PUBLICATIONS. Monthly newsletter. Lists new acquisitions.

LIBRARY OF CONGRESS *See* D12, D13

ELI LILLY AND COMPANY *See* F18

E25. MEDICAL COLLEGE OF WISCONSIN—MEDICAL-DENTAL LIBRARY, 560 N. 16 St., Milwaukee, Wisc. 53233. *Tel:* (414) 272-5450. Bessie A. Stein, Library Dir.

PURPOSE. To serve the students and faculty of the Medical College of Wisconsin and Marquette University School of Dentistry, hospitals in southeastern Wisconsin, and health professionals. *Specialization:* biomedicine and dentistry.
SPECIAL INFORMATION SERVICES. MEDLINE, TOXLINE, CHEMCON, ERIC, CAIN.
PUBLICATIONS. Newsletter, recent acquisitions, serials list.
INQUIRY ADDRESS. Reference Section, Medical College of Wisconsin, Medical-Dental Library, 560 N. 16 St., Milwaukee, Wisc, 53233. *Tel:* (414) 272-5450, ext. 240.

MEDICAL LIBRARY ASSOCIATION *See* A145

E26. THE MEDICAL LIBRARY CENTER OF NEW YORK, 17 E. 102 St., New York, N.Y. 10029. *Tel:* (212) 427-1630. Jean K. Miller, Dir.

PURPOSE. To maintain collection of periodicals and books for shared use of member libraries. *Specialization:* medical library.

MEMBERSHIP. *Requirements:* must be institution maintaining library for health sciences in New York metropolitan area. Operating funds derived from membership fees.

SPECIAL INFORMATION SERVICES. Foreign medical theses.

PUBLICATIONS. *Union Catalog of Medical Periodicals,* includes over 28,000 periodicals and serials and holdings of 92 New York City area libraries. Payment not required with order.

NATIONAL AGRICULTURAL LIBRARY *See* D14

NATIONAL ASSOCIATION OF HOSPITAL PURCHASING MANAGEMENT *See* A156

NATIONAL EASTER SEAL SOCIETY *See* A160

E27. NATIONAL INFORMATION CENTER FOR EDUCATIONAL MEDIA (NICEM), University of Southern California, Los Angeles, Calif. 90007. *Tel:* (213) 746-6681. Dr. Tom Risner, Dir.

PURPOSE. Custom computerized cataloging for audiovisual centers, libraries, colleges, universities, and media centers. Catalogs created are of client's holdings in all media. *Specialization:* indexes on nonbook educational media.

SPECIAL INFORMATION SERVICES. Automated book cataloging on nonbook educational material.

PUBLICATIONS. Lively brochure outlining NICEM's "Rx for AV Catalog Headaches." Application form for becoming client of custom cataloging service is included. Also brochure on nonprint information service, with book and microfiche updating. Lists indexes which each have several thousand entries in all media; also editions on producers and distributors. Multimedia indexes. Payment required with order.

NATIONAL LIBRARY OF MEDICINE *See* D20

NATIONAL SOCIETY FOR THE PREVENTION OF BLINDNESS *See* A174

E28. NATIONAL TECHNICAL INFORMATION SERVICE, U.S. Department of Commerce, Springfield, Va. 22161.*

PURPOSE. "To gather, organize, and communicate U.S. government-sponsored research and other unique technical information." *Specialization:* technical information.

PUBLICATIONS. The nation's largest publisher, NTIS adds 60,000 new titles each year to its stock. All are available in paper copy or microfiche. Some computer tapes are available. Materials of interest to health are numerous. *Health Planning* newsletter (weekly, $40) is new. A number of bibliographies available. One of their most important publications is *Medical Subject Headings* ($7.25), the National Library of Medicine subject heading list. Many publications formerly available from the Government Printing Office are now NTIS publications. Catalog available. Payment required with order, but American Express card may be used or an advance deposit account.

E29. NEW YORK ACADEMY OF MEDICINE, LIBRARY, 2 E. 103 St., New York, N.Y. 10029. *Tel:* (212) 876-8200. Alfred N. Brandon, Librarian.

PURPOSE. An academy founded in 1847 to promote public health, research, medical education, and to insure high standards in the medical professions. The library is an integral branch of the academy. *Specialization:* foreign monographs, textbooks, encyclopedias, indexes, bibliography, biography, history, Americana, portraits of physicians.
MEMBERSHIP. *Requirements:* members are elected by the fellowship. Library and information services open to all. Borrowing privileges extended to fellows of the academy and library subscribers.
SPECIAL INFORMATION SERVICES. *Special collections:* Malloch Rare Book and History of Medicine Room contains medical references, many classics, histories. Edwin Smith surgical papyrus dates from 2000 B.C.
PUBLICATIONS. Information on history of the academy and functions and guide to library. Academy offers publications in medicine from various publishers. Special series in history of medicine includes reprints of texts dating back to 1713. Reknown Library, open to the public, has over 400,000 volumes, 170,000 pamphlets, 5,400 periodical titles, and 500 annual reports in the field of medicine. Files include government publications and data on vital statistics. Catalogs to these immense resources, available from G. K. Hall, Boston, reproduce library's author and subject catalogs, and portrait, illustration, and biographies catalogs.

E30. NORTHWESTERN UNIVERSITY DENTAL SCHOOL LIBRARY, 311 E. Chicago Ave., Chicago, Ill. 60611. *Tel:* (312) 649-8332. Minnie Orfanos, Librarian.

PURPOSE. To support curriculum, teaching program, and research of Northwestern University Dental School. *Specialization:* dentistry.
SPECIAL INFORMATION SERVICES. *Special collections:* rare books on dentistry; special historical anesthesia collection.
PUBLICATIONS. Acquisitions lists, audiovisual lists. Payment not required with order.

E31. OHIO STATE UNIVERSITY HEALTH SCIENCES LIBRARY, 376 W. Tenth Ave., Columbus, Ohio 43210. *Tel:* (614) 422-8482.

PURPOSE. To provide health sciences materials to the medical complex of the Ohio State University—the Colleges of Medicine, Dentistry, and Optometry and the Schools of Nursing and Allied Medical Professions.
SPECIAL INFORMATION SERVICES. Medical reference, MEDLINE.

E32. OHIO STATE UNIVERSITY PHARMACY LIBRARY, 500 W. 12 Ave., Columbus, Ohio 43210. *Tel:* (614) 422-8026. Virginia B. Hall, Librarian.

PURPOSE. To serve the students and faculty of Ohio State University College of Pharmacy. (Services restricted to faculty in Ohio colleges, students and faculty of the university, and libraries [for interlibrary loans].) *Specialization:* pharmacology.

SPECIAL INFORMATION SERVICES. *Special collections:* pharmacy, pharmacology, medicinal chemistry, pharmaceutics, and pharmacy administration.
PUBLICATIONS. Six slide-tapes on use of library and its materials for beginning students. Orients user to card catalog, indexes, and search for literature. Free loan.

POPULATION REFERENCE BUREAU *See* A186

REHABILITATION SERVICES ADMINISTRATION *See* D25

E33. RUSH MEDICAL COLLEGE LIBRARY, 1758 W. Harrison St., Chicago, Ill. 60612. *Tel:* (312) 942-5950. William Kona, Dir.

PURPOSE. To serve the Medical College, Nursing College, and allied health institutions. Affiliated with Rush-Presbyterian-St. Luke's Medical Center.
PUBLICATIONS. Multimedia catalog.

E34. ST. PAUL PUBLIC LIBRARY, 90 W. Fourth St., St. Paul, Minn. 55102. *Tel:* (612) 224-3383. Richard T. Hemming, Acquisitions Librarian.

PURPOSE. A public library for the populace of St. Paul and the surrounding metropolitan area. (Services restricted to St. Paul residents or residents of area with contractual agreement with St. Paul.) *Specialization:* bibliographies.
PUBLICATIONS. Large-print catalogs; Indian culture and life publications list; career guide list includes medical careers; library newsletter; list of women's studies, including books on medical subjects for women—sex, menstruation, contraception.

E35. STANFORD UNIVERSITY MEDICAL CENTER—LANE MEDICAL LIBRARY, Stanford, Calif. 94305. *Tel:* (415) 497-7113. Peter Stangl, Dir.

PURPOSE. To provide literature and information services for medical personnel, students, and all the Stanford community.
MEMBERSHIP. Personal memberships available.
PUBLICATIONS. Audiotapes for in-library use being prepared.
SPECIAL INFORMATION SERVICES. MEDLINE, DIALOG. *Special collections:* history of medicine; ophthalmology; and historical collection of medical journals.

STATE OF MAINE DEPARTMENT OF HEALTH AND WELFARE *See* D28

E36. STATE UNIVERSITY OF NEW YORK (SUNY) BIOMEDICAL COMMUNICATION NETWORK, 99 Washington Ave., Albany, N.Y. 12210. *Tel:* (518) 474-1771.

PURPOSE. To provide on-line access to bibliographic data bases in the sciences to academic or research institutions via nonprofit regional network. (Services restricted to academic or government research institutions.)
MEMBERSHIP. *Requirements:* restricted to academic institutions. Annual fixed fee for unlimited access (about $7,200/yr.).
SPECIAL INFORMATION SERVICES. Computerized files (used by 33 institutions in ten states) include MEDLARS, ERIC, Psychological Abstracts, and (experimentally) Biological Abstracts.

INQUIRY ADDRESS. Central Office Computer Center, State University of New York (SUNY) Biomedical Communications Network, 99 Washington Ave., Albany, N.Y. 12210. *Tel:* (518) 474-1771.

E37. STATE UNIVERSITY OF NEW YORK AT STONY BROOK—HEALTH SCIENCES LIBRARY/HEALTH SCIENCES CENTER, Box 66, East Setauket, N.Y. 11733. *Tel:* (516) 444-2515. Mrs. Mary Winkels, Dir.

PURPOSE. To serve the faculty, staff, and students of the Health Sciences Center and the university community and all persons in Nassau and Suffolk counties involved in health-care delivery. (Services restricted to individuals in health-care delivery.)
SPECIAL INFORMATION SERVICES. SUNY Biomedical Communication Network, MEDLINE, CATLINE, SERLINE, CANCERLINE, TOXLINE. *Special collections:* allied health professions, basic health sciences, dental medicine, nursing, medicine, podiatric medicine, and social welfare.

E38. UNIVERSITY OF CALIFORNIA (BERKELEY)—EDUCATION/PSYCHOLOGY LIBRARY, 2600 Tolman Hall, Berkeley, Calif. 94720. *Tel:* (415) 642-4208. Margaret Stern, Head Librarian.

PURPOSE. To collect, maintain, and make available publications in education, psychology, and related fields to meet teaching and research needs of faculty, students, and the community at large. (Open to public, but circulation for home use requires university card or fee card.) *Specialization:* education and psychology.
SPECIAL INFORMATION SERVICES. *Special collections:* health education and mental health (including multimedia catalog).

E39. UNIVERSITY OF CALIFORNIA (SAN FRANCISCO), Langley Porter Neuropsychiatric Institute Library, 401 Parnassus Ave., San Francisco, Calif. 94143. *Tel:* (415) 681-8080, ext. 380. Edwarda Adams, Librarian.

PURPOSE. To supply information needs of the institute staff, students, and trainees. Porter Institute is an academic research and teaching hospital. (Services restricted to Porter Institute staff, students, and trainees.) *Specialization:* neuropsychiatry.
SPECIAL INFORMATION SERVICES. *Special collections:* psychiatry, psychoanalysis, clinical psychology, and allied fields (about 15,000 volumes).

E40. UNIVERSITY OF CALIFORNIA (SAN FRANCISCO), Library, San Francisco, Calif. 94143. *Tel:* (415) 666-2334. Mrs. Jeanette G. Yeazell, University Librarian.

PURPOSE. To provide library services to faculty, students, and staff of the university and to other qualified health professionals. *Specialization:* health sciences (380,000 volumes).
SPECIAL INFORMATION SERVICES. *Special collections:* history of health sciences.

E41. UNIVERSITY OF CONNECTICUT HEALTH CENTER, Lyman Maynard Stowe Library, Farmington, Conn. 06032. *Tel:* (203) 674-2840.

PURPOSE. To serve the information needs of the Health Center and health professionals in Connecticut. *Specialization:* medicine, dentistry, nursing, and allied health fields.

SPECIAL INFORMATION SERVICES. ILL, NLM data bases; reference service extended to other libraries, health professionals, and Connecticut residents. *Special collections:* collection of 1,847 audiovisuals in health sciences available for loan through ILL and by special arrangement.

PUBLICATIONS. *New Acquisitions* (monthly); *Serials Holdings* (annual); *Connecticut Audio-Visual Union List* (annual).

E42. UNIVERSITY OF HAWAII—SCHOOL OF PUBLIC HEALTH, 1960 East West Rd., Library, D-207, Honolulu, Hawaii 96822. *Tel:* (808) 948-8666. Margaret C. Lane, Librarian.

PURPOSE. To serve students, staff, and faculty of the School of Public Health, and others in the community in need of specialized public health information. *Specialization:* health administration, education, personal health services, public health sciences, and international health, with emphasis on Asia and the Pacific.

SPECIAL INFORMATION SERVICES. Twenty thousand microfiche on health services administration.

PUBLICATIONS. *Pacific Health* (annual); other items at irregular intervals. *Pacific Health* available on exchange. Payment not required with order.

E43. UNIVERSITY OF IOWA, HEALTH SCIENCES LIBRARY, Iowa City, Iowa 52242. *Tel:* (319) 353-5382. Dr. Leslie Dunlap, Dean, University Libraries.

PUPROSE. To serve the health-care community at the University of Iowa in medicine, dentistry, pharmacy, speech pathology, audiology, nursing, and hospital and health administration. Also serves as major health sciences resource center for the state of Iowa. (Services restricted to members of health-care field in state of Iowa.) *Specialization:* health sciences.

PUBLICATIONS. *The Heirs of Hippocrates*, ed. Frank Hanlin—catalog of John Martin Rare Book Room Collection—available only to members of Friends of the Library.

SPECIAL INFORMATION SERVICES. MEDLINE, telephoned reference inquiries. *Special collections:* John Martin Rare Book Collection—rare and valuable historical books, including first edition of Vesalius.

E44. UNIVERSITY OF MICHIGAN, CHEMISTRY-PHARMACY LIBRARY, 2200 Chemistry Building, Ann Arbor, Mich. 48104. *Tel:* (313) 764-7337. Margaret Z. Jones, Librarian.

PURPOSE. To provide bibliographical and physical access to materials in fields of chemistry and pharmacy. (Services primarily for students and staff of the university.)

SPECIAL INFORMATION SERVICES. *Special collections:* History of Pharmacy (about 125 titles including some early works), U.S. Pharmacopoeias and Formularies.

PUBLICATIONS. Bibliographies for student use.

E45. UNIVERSITY OF MICHIGAN—PUBLIC HEALTH LIBRARY, Ann Arbor, Mich. 48104. *Tel:* (313) 764-5473. L. C. Yu, Head.

PURPOSE. To support the School of Public Health's graduate teaching curriculum and its faculty members' research activities. *Specialization:* comprehensive collections in public health, health economics, community health services, biostatistics, and several other health fields. 30,000 monographs; 500 journal titles.

SPECIAL INFORMATION SERVICES. *Special collections:* Medical care organization, hospital administration, maternal and child health, and population planning.

E46. UNIVERSITY OF MISSOURI—COLUMBIA MEDICAL LIBRARY, M210 Medical Center, Columbia, Mo. 65201. *Tel:* (314) 882-8086. Dean Schmidt, Librarian.

PURPOSE. To provide informational materials to meet educational, research, and patient care needs of the University of Missouri-Columbia Medical Center. (Services offered primarily to faculty, students, and staff of the university; secondarily to health practitioners in Missouri.)

SPECIAL INFORMATION SERVICES. MEDLINE, reference, and consultation.

E47. UNIVERSITY OF NEBRASKA MEDICAL CENTER—LIBRARY OF MEDICINE, 42 St. and Dewey Ave., Omaha, Nebr. 68105. *Tel:* (402) 541-4006. David Bishop, Dir.

PURPOSE. To provide library services to the students, faculty, and staff of the university, to health professionals in Nebraska, and throughout seven-state midcontinental region. (Services restricted to professionals in health and allied fields.) *Specialization:* medical library of University of Nebraska Medical Center.

SPECIAL INFORMATION SERVICES. Includes on-line computer-based bibliographies (MEDLINE) and Learning Resources Center (audiovisuals) for curriculum support. Administrative headquarters for Midcontinental Regional Medical Library Program. *Special collections:* Health services administration collection, AAMC/GPR archive, history of Nebraska medicine.

PUBLICATIONS. *Health Services Administration Collection Bibliography* listing materials available to health service professionals in Nebraska, Colorado, Kansas, Missouri, South Dakota, Utah, and Wyoming. Large selection of books on hospital administration; other areas of health care also covered. Dozens of periodicals, audiocassettes also available.

INQUIRY ADDRESSES. Reference Department, Library of Medicine, (402) 541-4006. Midcontinental Regional Medical Library, (402) 541-4646. Both at University of Nebraska Medical Center, Library of Medicine, 42 St. and Dewey Ave., Omaha, Nebr. 68105.

E48. UNIVERSITY OF NEW MEXICO HEALTH SCIENCES LIBRARY, North Campus, Albuquerque, N.M. 87131. *Tel:* (505) 277-2311. Dr. Robert T. Divett, Librarian.

PURPOSE. To support the teaching and research efforts of the School of Medicine, the College of Nursing, the College of Pharmacy, and the Allied Health Programs of the University of New Mexico, and to provide statewide services, including document copying and loans, reference service, and consultation with faculty members through the TALON Regional Medical Library Program. (Services restricted to health

science professionals in New Mexico or to out-of-state health sciences personnel through their regional medical libraries.)
SPECIAL INFORMATION SERVICES. Document copying and loans, reference service, and consultation with faculty members.
INQUIRY ADDRESS. Interlibrary Loan Section, University of New Mexico Health Sciences Library, North Campus, Albuquerque, N.M. 87131. *Tel:* (505) 277-2311.

E49. UNIVERSITY OF OREGON HEALTH SCIENCES LIBRARY, 3181 S.W. Sam Jackson Park Rd., Portland, Oreg. 97201. *Tel:* (503) 225-8026. James E. Morgan, Director of Libraries.

PURPOSE. To provide informational services to faculty and students of University of Oregon Health Sciences Center, and to provide resource library services to health professionals in Oregon, when desired materials are unavailable at local level. (Services generally restricted to health sciences professionals.)
SPECIAL INFORMATION SERVICES. MEDLINE and other MEDLARS data bases; plans in effect for adding Lockheed and SDC data bases. *Special collections:* Pacific Northwest Regional Collection dealing with physicians, nurses, and events of interest medically in Washington and Oregon.

E50. UNIVERSITY OF PITTSBURGH—MAURICE AND LAURA FALK LIBRARY OF THE HEALTH PROFESSIONS, DeSoto and Terrace St., Pittsburgh, Pa. 15261. *Tel:* (412) 624-2520.

PURPOSE. To support the curricula of the health professions courses: medicine, dentistry, nursing, public health, and pharmacy. (Services restricted to scholars pursuing research in history of the health sciences and health professions.) *Specialization:* health sciences and health professions.
SPECIAL INFORMATION SERVICES. MEDLINE, CATLINE, and SERLINE. *Special collections:* nursing and historical collections, latter containing material relating to all health sciences.
PUBLICATIONS. Handbook on use of library and one on the Historical Collection. *Recent Acquisitions* (monthly), *Library Bulletin* (occasional), and *Union List of Serials.* Payment not required with order.

E51. UNIVERSITY OF SOUTH DAKOTA SCHOOL OF MEDICINE—HEALTH SCIENCE LIBRARY, Vermillion, S.D. 57069. *Tel:* (605) 677-5348. Patrick Brennan, Dir.

PURPOSE. To service professional and paraprofessional health care in South Dakota. *Specialization:* health sciences.
SPECIAL INFORMATION SERVICES. MEDLINE, SIDLINE, SERLINE, CATLINE, and TOXLINE at a charge for each search. *Special collection:* growing audiovisual collection in support of clinical faculty for third- and fourth-year medical students.
PUBLICATIONS. Library handbook.

E52. UNIVERSITY OF TEXAS CANCER CENTER, M. D. Anderson Hospital and Tumor Institute, Library, 6723 Bertner Dr., Houston, Tex. 77025. *Tel:* (713) 792-2282. Marie Harvin, Research Medical Librarian.

PURPOSE. To provide literature and information support for faculty, staff, and trainees at 300-bed cancer hospital with large cancer research program and extensive postgraduate educational activities. (Services restricted to physicians, dentists, and other allied health personnel.) *Specialization:* neoplastic disease, diagnosis and treatment of cancer, and cancer research.
SPECIAL INFORMATION SERVICES. MEDLINE and CANCERLINE. Manually compiled bibliographies, as well as computerized current articles on neoplasia.
PUBLICATIONS. *Current Articles on Neoplasia,* 36-page weekly bibliography. Approximately 900 journals represented. Free to practitioners, investigators, scientific organizations, and libraries. *Year Book of Cancer* reviews most significant articles.

E53. UNIVERSITY OF UTAH—SPENCER S. ECCLES MEDICAL SCIENCES LIBRARY, Salt Lake City, Utah 84112. *Tel:* (801) 581-8771. Priscilla M. Mayden, Library Dir.

PURPOSE. To serve the University of Utah's colleges of the Health Science Complex—Medicine, Nursing, Pharmacy, and Health. (Services restricted to university's staff and faculty.) *Specialization:* medical sciences.
SPECIAL INFORMATION SERVICES. MEDLINE, TOXLINE/CHEMLINE, CANCERLINE, CATLINE, SERLINE, AVLINE, ERIC, MATRIX, several other data bases from Systems Development Corporation and Lockheed, plus ASCA current awareness service.

E54. UNIVERSITY OF VERMONT—CHARLES A. DANA MEDICAL LIBRARY, Burlington, Vt. 05401. *Tel:* (802) 656-2200. Ellen Gillies, Medical Librarian.

PURPOSE. To acquire, store, and disseminate health science information for use of students and faculty of Division of Health Sciences and staff of Medical Center Hospital of Vermont.

E55. VANDERBILT UNIVERSITY MEDICAL CENTER LIBRARY, Nashville, Tenn. 37232. *Tel:* (615) 322-2292. T. Mark Hodges, Dir.

PURPOSE. A primary information resource for professional personnel and students in medicine, nursing, and allied sciences at Vanderbilt University. (Services restricted to professional personnel and students at Vanderbilt University, Peabody and Scarritt colleges, and Nashville Academy of Medicine.) *Specialization:* medical library.
SPECIAL INFORMATION SERVICES. MEDLINE. *Special collections:* history of medicine collection.
PUBLICATIONS. Free newsletter and guide to library.
INQUIRY ADDRESS. Reference and Research Services, Vanderbilt University Medical Center Library, Nashville, Tenn. 37232. *Tel:* (615) 322-2292.

E56. WASHINGTON UNIVERSITY SCHOOL OF MEDICINE LIBRARY, 4580 Scott Ave., St. Louis, Mo. 63110. *Tel:* (314) 454-3711. Dr. Estelle Brodman, Librarian.

PURPOSE. To serve library needs of Washington University School of Medicine and

Medical Center. (Services restricted to health personnel affiliated with Washington University Medical Center.) *Specialization:* medicine and health sciences.

SPECIAL INFORMATION SERVICES. ERIC, CAIN, CHEMCON, TOXLINE, NTIS, MEDLINE, and CAI.

PUBLICATIONS. Guides to use of library, archives, and computerized information systems. Audiotapes, indexes. Payment not required with order.

INQUIRY ADDRESS. Reference Department, Washington University School of Medicine Library, 4580 Scott Ave., St. Louis, Mo. 63110. *Tel:* (314) 454-3711.

E57. YALE MEDICAL LIBRARY, 333 Cedar St., New Haven, Conn. 06510.* *Tel:* (203) 436-4784. Stanley D. Truelson, Jr., Librarian.

PURPOSE. To serve the Yale community and provide reference service to health professionals in the state through their hospital libraries.

PUBLICATIONS. A series of guides to searching the literature are available for a small fee.

F

Pharmaceutical
and Other
Companies

F1. ABBOTT LABORATORIES, Public Affairs, D-383, Abbott Park, North Chicago, Ill. 60064. *Tel:* (312) 688-3930. Edward J. Ledder, Pres. and Chief Executive Officer.

PURPOSE. A manufacturer of health-care products, principally prescription pharmaceuticals, hospital products, diagnostic products, and instrumentation. *Specialization:* medical films and publications for professional audiences.
PUBLICATIONS. Medical subjects generally for professional audiences. Diagnostic atlases and instructional aids, films on diagnosis, internal medicine, heart attacks, surgery, patient education, and mental illness; majority are instructional films, but some are features with professional actors. Three films available to lay audiences; publications for lay readers on understanding drugs, hay fever, rheumatic fever, venereal disease, and hepatitis. Up to 50 of these available without charge. Payment required with order for publications that carry charges; not required with film rental order.

F2. ASTRA PHARMACEUTICAL PRODUCTS, INC., Audiovisual Communications, Neponset St., Worcester, Mass. 01606.* *Tel:* (617) 852-6351.

PURPOSE. A drug manufacturer, offering free-loan films to professionals. *Specialization:* free-loan films.
PUBLICATIONS. 16mm sound-color films for physicians, dentists, hospitals, professional societies, and teaching institutions. Thirty on medical technique and eight on dentistry from various producers.

F3. AYERST LABORATORIES, Medical Information Service, 685 Third Ave., New York, N.Y. 10017.*

PURPOSE. To offer free-loan films to medical professionals for specialized audiences. *Specialization:* free-loan films.
PUBLICATIONS. Films listed in loose-leaf catalog. Medical procedures and product information are covered.

F4. BAUSCH AND LOMB, 1400 N. Goodman St., Rochester, N.Y. 14602.

PURPOSE. A manufacturer of optical devices and safety products. *Specialization:* eye safety and microscopy.
PUBLICATIONS. Free-loan films on eye safety and use of B&L microscopes. Films illustrate importance of eye protection at work, aspects of vision and eye care, technique of microscopy, and principles of microscope use for high school biology students.

F5. BECTON/DICKINSON, Rutherford, N.J. 07070. *Tel:* (201) 939-9000. Wesley J. Howe, Pres.

PURPOSE. A manufacturer of laboratory equipment and pharmaceutical devices. *Specialization:* manufacturing of medical apparatus.
PUBLICATIONS. Five 16mm color films available for free rental. Topics include careers in bacteriology, parental injection techniques, intravenous infusion, and use of company's "Vacutainer" apparatus and culture tubes.

F6. BURROUGHS WELLCOME COMPANY, Research, Triangle Park, N.C. 27709.*

PURPOSE. A pharmaceuticals and medical supplies manufacturer. *Specialization:* free-loan films.
PUBLICATIONS. List of 23 free-loan films for medical professionals. Slide show "Catheter Care" on preventing infection in and around catheter tubes.

F7. CAMPBELL SOUP COMPANY, Department 630 J, Camden, N.J. 08101.*

PURPOSE. A food manufacturer, offering pamphlets to doctors for educating and counseling patients. *Specialization:* patient education.
PUBLICATIONS. Teaching aids include slides accompanied by syllabi, covering vitamins, digestion, aging, maternal nutrition, and diabetes. Payment not required with order.

F8. CARNATION RESEARCH LABORATORIES, 8015 Van Nuys Blvd., Van Nuys, Calif. 91412. *Tel:* 787-7820. J. M. McIntire, Gen. Mgr.

PURPOSE. Research on foods. (Services restricted to lab employees.)
SPECIAL INFORMATION SERVICES. Literature searches.

F9. CAROLINA BIOLOGICAL SUPPLY COMPANY, 2700 York Rd., Burlington, N.C. 27215. *Tel:* (919) 584-0381. Thomas E. Powell, Jr., Pres.

PURPOSE. To supply biological materials to schools and research. *Specialization:* life sciences.

PUBLICATIONS. "Discoveries of Early Man" series of plastic anthropoidal skull models, along with books on the subject. *Oxford Biology Readers:* general principles of biological study, along with birth control, mammalian hearts and lungs, evolution, metamorphosis; about 50 titles in series, in format of booklets of about 20 pages (illustrated). *Carolina Tips* (monthly), newsletter. *Catalog of Biological Materials* runs to 550 pages—living animals and plants, models, preserved specimens, microscope slides, 2 × 2 slides, offprints, filmstrips, charts, laboratory media—all accessories for biological study available; this is the Sears and Roebuck of the biology world.

F10. CIBA MEDICAL EDUCATION DIVISION, CIBA-GEIGY Corporation, 556 Morris Ave., Summit, N.J. 07901. *Tel:* (201) 277-5477. Robert Luciano, Pres.

PURPOSE. A pharmaceutical manufacturer publishing on a nonprofit basis medical illustrations for the medical profession. *Specialization:* anatomy, physiology, and pathology.
PUBLICATIONS. *CIBA Collection of Medical Illustrations* is an eight-volume set of anatomical paintings by Frank Netter, M.D., sample pages shown in catalog. An authoritative and detailed guide to anatomy and diagnosis. Also 2,200 medical illustrations on 35mm slides by Netter and others. Separate catalog for 35mm slides. Payment required with order.

F11. COOK-WAITE LABORATORIES, INC., Division of Professional Services, 90 Park Ave., New York, N.Y. 10016.* J. W. Lee, D.D.S., Vice-Pres.

PURPOSE. An industrial concern providing free-loan films on dentistry to professionals. *Specialization:* dentistry.
PUBLICATIONS. Films on medication, anesthesia, and patient comfort for dental schools, professional societies, study clubs, and other professional groups and teaching institutions.

F12. DENAR CORPORATION, 2020 Howell Ave., Anaheim, Calif. 92806. *Tel:* (714) 634-3344. Ralph Stern, Pres.

PURPOSE. To manufacture precision occlusal instrumentation for use in dentistry and promote occlusal education in this field. *Specialization:* dental occlusion.
PUBLICATIONS. Books, pamphlets, slides, audiotapes, videotapes, and periodicals. Several lab and technique manuals ($10–$25); a number of slide series like "Occlusion" slide series, "Full Denture" slide series ($45 each set); Occlusial Examination Forms ($11.25); and a movie, *Principles of Occlusion,* which rents for $14.75 a week. Deposit required with large instrumentation order.

F13. DUNLAP AND ASSOCIATES, INC., One Parkland Dr., Darien, Conn. 06820. *Tel:* (203) 655-3971. Jack W. Dunlap, Pres. and Chmn. of the Board.

PURPOSE. A research consultant in health services planning, analysis, and evaluation (EMS, drug and alcohol abuse programs, and highway safety).

F14. EATON MEDICAL FILM LIBRARY, Eaton Laboratories Division, Norwich Pharmaceutical Company, Norwich, N.Y. 13815.*

PURPOSE. Pharmaceutical maker offering free-loan films to professionals. *Specialization:* medical films.
PUBLICATIONS. Catalog of films available for free loan through local Eaton representative or directly from the library. Most medical specialties covered. Other multimedia programs.

F15. EMPLOYERS INSURANCE OF WAUSAU, Special Services Department, Wausau, Wisc. 54401.* *Tel:* (715) 842-6544.

PURPOSE. An insurance company offering safety and health materials to policyholders. *Specialization:* health and safety.
PUBLICATIONS. Charts, forms, literature, posters, and films. 16mm films on safety management and occupational safety are loaned free to policyholders.

F16. GEIGY PHARMACEUTICALS, Ardsley, N.Y. 10502.* Frederick E. Muster, Dir. of Medical Services.

PURPOSE. A pharmaceuticals company offering free-loan films to professionals. *Specialization:* medical films.
PUBLICATIONS. Films loaned without charge for showings to medical or scientific audiences.16mm films concerned with particular diseases, management of practice, and psychiatry. Catalog lists about 20 films (with abstracts).

F17. JOHNSON AND JOHNSON, 501 George St., New Brunswick, N.J. 08903. Richard B. Sellars, Chief Executive Officer.

PURPOSE. *Specialization:* baby care and personal care.
PUBLICATIONS. Booklets on baby care, films on bringing up baby (free loan), and booklets and film on personal hygiene for teenagers. Up to 200 free booklets for classroom use.

F18. ELI LILLY AND COMPANY, 307 E. McCarty St., Indianapolis, Ind. 46206. *Tel:* (317) 261-3263. R. D. Wood, Chmn. of the Board.

PURPOSE. Pharmaceuticals manufacturer with educational resources library. (Some services restricted to medical professionals.) *Specialization:* medical education and public relations information.
PUBLICATIONS. Materials in all media. *General Interests* catalog lists films and slide sets on health, nutrition, and drugs. Pharmacy catalog includes diagnosis, surgery, patient care, internal medicine, and pharmacology. Educational Resources Program with films and slides primarily for medical professionals and students; also lists videotapes, monographs, and brochures. Covers diagnosis and treatment of specific ailments, including internal medicine, dermatology, and surgery. Payment not required with order.
INQUIRY ADDRESS. Miss Annetta I. Proctor, Eli Lilly and Company, 307 E. McCarty St., Indianapolis, Ind. 46206. *Tel:* (317) 261-2028.

F19. MILTON ROY COMPANY, OPHTHALMIC GROUP, Box 1899, Sarasota, Fla. 33578. *Tel:* (813) 755-1526. Raleigh S. Althisar, Sr., Pres.

PURPOSE. A manufacturer and distributor of prescription contact lenses, optical services (eyeglass lenses and frames), and ophthalmic solutions and instruments. *Specialization:* ophthalmic supplies and services.
PUBLICATIONS. Mostly of interest to ophthalmologists, optometrists, opticians, and other practitioners. Information on contacts and other products. Pamphlets on cleaning and insertion for wearers of contacts. Payment not required with order.
INQUIRY ADDRESS. Miss M. Fromow, Advertising Mgr., Milton Roy Company, Ophthalmic Group, Box 1899, Sarasota, Fla. 33578. *Tel:* (813) 755-1526.

F20. PERSONAL PRODUCTS COMPANY, Milltown, N.J. 08850. Arlene Krupinski, Mgr., Consumer Information Center.

PURPOSE. A manufacturer of feminine hygiene products and distributor of information on menstruation and female development. *Specialization:* feminine hygiene.
PUBLICATIONS. Resource materials for pre-teenage, teenager, and young women include pamphlets on growing up, manual for mothers on advising daughters on menstruation, film *Naturally a Girl* for free loan in English and Spanish, and booklet telling boys about girls growing up. Phono record, braille, and large print versions covering same areas. Teacher's guide to feminine hygiene. Payment required with order.

PHARMACEUTICALS MANUFACTURERS ASSOCIATION *See* A181

F21. A. H. ROBINS COMPANY, Medical Film Service Department, 1407 Cummings Dr., Richmond, Va. 23220.*

PURPOSE. A pharmaceuticals company with free-loan film plan. *Specialization:* pharmaceuticals.
PUBLICATIONS. List of 14 films for both general and professional audiences. Emphasis on use of pharmaceuticals.

F22. ROCHE FILM LIBRARY, c/o Association-Sterling Films, Inc., 600 Grand Ave., Ridgefield, N.J. 07657.*

PURPOSE. A division of Hoffman-LaRoche Pharmaceuticals, loaning free films to professionals. *Specialization:* free-loan films.
PUBLICATIONS. "Frontiers of Psychiatry" series of ten films (some on medicolegal problems).

F23. ROCOM, Box 270, Nutley, N.J. 07110.* *Tel:* (201) 235-4875.

PURPOSE. A division of Hoffman-LaRoche Pharmaceuticals, selling materials for management of medical practices. *Specialization:* medical management and administration.
PUBLICATIONS. Medical Management System offered, in form of records forms, case history questionnaires (English and Spanish), flow charts, and files for indexes. *Patient Health Guide* booklets. Minimum order $25. Payment not required with order.

F24. ROERIG DIVISION FILM LIBRARY, Pfizer Pharmaceuticals, New York, N.Y. 10017.*

PURPOSE. A pharmaceuticals company with instructional films for free loan to medical professionals. *Specialization:* free-loan films.
PUBLICATIONS. Many films on psychiatry—schizophrenia, manic-depressive states, etc.

F25. ROSS AUDIO VISUAL LIBRARY, Ross Laboratories, Division of Abbott Laboratories USA, 625 Cleveland Ave., Columbus, Ohio 43216.*

PURPOSE. A pharmaceuticals company, loaning free films for medical professionals and general public. *Specialization:* free-loan films.
PUBLICATIONS. Films emphasize child care, maternal and child health, and neonatology for professionals. For lay audiences, films available touch on breast feeding, nutrition for babies, and similar topics. Films may be purchased.

F26. SANDOZ PHARMACEUTICALS, Medical Film Library, East Hanover, N.J. 07936.*

PURPOSE. A pharmaceuticals manufacturer, producer of free-loan films for medical professionals. *Specialization:* films for medical professionals.
PUBLICATIONS. Films on 16mm stock and in super-8 cartridges for showings to medical students, professionals, and professional groups. Large psychiatry selection; also pediatrics, obstetrics, hematology, and other fields.

F27. SCHERING PROFESSIONAL FILM LIBRARY, Eastern Film Distribution Center, c/o Association Films, Inc., 600 Grand Ave., Ridgefield, N.J. 07657.*

PURPOSE. To distribute free-loan instructional films for medical and paramedical groups. *Specialization:* free-loan medical films.
PUBLICATIONS. Thirty-page pamphlet lists allergy, health education (many for lay audiences), neurology, surgery, veterinary medicine, along with large dermatology section.

F28. G. D. SEARLE AND COMPANY, Box 5110, Chicago, Ill. 60680.*

PURPOSE. *Specialization:* medical films.
PUBLICATIONS. Free-loan films for medical professionals.

F29. SHELL FILM LIBRARY, 1433 Sadlier Circle West Dr., Indianapolis, Ind. 46239.* *Tel:* (317) 291-7440.

PURPOSE. A multinational petroleum producer offering free-loan educational films to schools and organizations. *Specialization:* free-loan films.
PUBLICATIONS. Booklet lists offerings, covers air pollution, pesticides, and world nutrition, as well as other topics.

F30. SMITH, KLINE, AND FRENCH LABORATORIES, 1500 Spring Garden St., Philadelphia, Pa. 19101.* *Tel:* (215) LO4-2400.

PURPOSE. A pharmaceuticals manufacturer producing health films. *Specialization:* films on medicine.

PUBLICATIONS. Films are for both general audience and medical professionals. Smith, Kline, and French offers list of its titles with respective distributors: medical techniques, nursing, medicosocial issues. Payment depends on particular distributor.

F31. SQUIBB MEDICAL FILMS, E. R. Squibb and Sons, Inc., Box 4000, Princeton, N.J. 08540.*

PURPOSE. A pharmaceuticals manufacturer offering free-loan teaching films to medical professionals. *Specialization:* free-loan medical teaching films.

PUBLICATIONS. One-hundred-page film catalog.

F32. SUNKIST GROWERS, INC., Consumer Service AV-72, Box 7888, Valley Annex, Van Nuys, Calif. 91409.*

PURPOSE. A produce grower, selling filmstrips to consumers. *Specialization:* nutrition for general audiences.

PUBLICATIONS. Filmstrips aimed at high schoolers and adults illustrating good nutrition. Payment not required with order.

F33. SYNTEX LABORATORIES, INC., Professional Services, 3401 Hillview Ave., Stanford Industrial Park, Palo Alto, Calif. 94304.*

PURPOSE. A pharmaceuticals manufacturer offering free-loan films and sound-filmstrips for professionals in the health field. *Specialization:* audiovisual materials for medical professionals.

PUBLICATIONS. Films and sound-filmstrips cover patient care, pharmaceuticals, and other areas.

F34. THE UPJOHN COMPANY, 7000 Portage Rd., Kalamazoo, Mich. 49001. *Tel:* (616) 382-4000. R. T. Parfet, Chmn. of the Board.

PURPOSE. A pharmaceuticals manufacturer with program to update medical and allied professions in new and clinically significant developments in medicine. (Services restricted to members of medical and allied professions.) *Specialization:* professional medical materials.

SPECIAL INFORMATION SERVICES. Medical Information and Review—for questions from professionals regarding Upjohn products.

PUBLICATIONS. Professional Film Library catalog of unbound descriptive pages. Dozens of films on exploratory surgery, cancer, microscopy, diabetes, transplants, and other topics. Also "Grand Rounds" with panels of distinguished physicians. "Mini texts" in 16mm or 8mm, listed in separate catalog, cover many of same subjects but with more emphasis on laser technology and internal examinations with fiber-optics. Also slides, audiotapes, and monographs. Two brief patient-oriented films on diabetes and insulin injection. Payment not required with order.

F35. WARD'S NATURAL SCIENCE ESTABLISHMENT, INC., Box 1712, Rochester, N.Y. 14603. *Tel:* (716) 467-8400. Robert D. Quigley, Vice-Pres.

PURPOSE. To provide biology and earth science specimen material, audiovisuals, and laboratory equipment and supplies for biology and earth sciences at high school–junior college levels. *Specialization:* educational materials for biology and earth sciences.

PUBLICATIONS. Thirty-six page catalog of films includes biology, chemistry, and general science. Slides and Solo-Learn Overhead transparencies. Payment not required with orders from institutions. Individuals should write for information.

INQUIRY ADDRESS. Ward's Customer Service, above address. Box 1712, Rochester, N.Y. 14603.

G

Publishers

G1. ACADEMIC PRESS, INC./GRUNE & STRATTON, INC., 111 Fifth Ave., New York, N.Y. 10003. *Tel:* (212) 741-6800. Charles Hutt, Pres.

PURPOSE. To publish scientific and medical books and journals. Both branches are divisions of Harcourt Brace Jovanovich. *Specialization:* Academic Press—biology, biochemistry and biomedicine, chemistry, physics and engineering, and behavioral and social sciences. Grune & Stratton—medicine, psychology and psychiatry, and special education.

PUBLICATIONS. Three free catalogs list Grune & Stratton publications in medicine and psychology; Academic Press works in biological sciences, and its volumes in medicine and biomedical sciences. Academic Press catalogs give precise descriptions of contents of their publications and are helpful in tracking down literature in specific fields or for choosing texts for advanced classes. Grune & Stratton catalog is somewhat less descriptive; it has smaller selection, with largest variety in field of psychiatry. Grune & Stratton also offers journals *Blood* (hematology), *Pediatric Surgery*, and ten other print periodicals. Two journals (*General Surgery* and *Ophthalmology*) come on audiotape cassettes. Payment not required with order.

G2. ADDISON-WESLEY PUBLISHING COMPANY, INC., Reading, Mass. 01867.

PURPOSE. To publish textbooks in science, health, psychology, and other areas of study.* *Specialization:* textbooks in science, health, and psychology.

PUBLICATIONS. Pamphlet-style listings for life sciences, physical sciences, health and physical education, and psychology—each listing about 25 pages—present detailed descriptions of available texts, most for college level. Basic biology, cell biology and biochemistry, genetics, physiology and neurobiology, physical biology, biological electronics, and instrumentation—series of original essays called *Modules in Biology*. Organic chemistry, human ecology, and physics for the life and health sciences, personality development, transactional analysis for students, and physiological psychology. Payment not required with order.

G3. AERO-MEDICAL CONSULTANTS, INC., 10912 Hamlin Blvd., Largo, Fla. 33540. *Tel:* (813) 596-2551. Eric James, Sales Mgr.

PURPOSE. Publisher. *Specialization:* aviation and medicine.
PUBLICATIONS. *Patient's Guide to Medicine, Advice to Folks Over Fifty*, and other books. Payment not required with order.

AIR POLLUTION TECHNICAL INFORMATION CENTER *See* E1

G4. ALDINE PUBLISHING COMPANY, 529 S. Wabash Ave., Chicago, Ill. 60605. *Tel:* (312) 939-5190. Lawrence I. Goldberg, Pres.

PURPOSE. To produce videotape programs and supplementary materials for the allied health fields and nursing. *Specialization:* videotapes on health and medicine.
PUBLICATIONS. Pamphlets describe wide variety of available programs. Topics include aphasia, radiologic technology (a program of 22 tapes treating skull exams, spine exams, extremities, thorax, and abdomen), and large selection in allied health. Latter includes human anatomy, anatomy lab, physiology, organic chemistry, nursing skills, pharmacology, and dental hygiene. Videotapes available in 3/4″ cassettes or 1/2″ reels. *Inner World of Aphasia*, 16mm film, can be purchased or rented. Payment not required with order.

G5. ALFRED ADLER INSTITUTE OF CHICAGO, INC., 110 S. Dearborn St., Suite 1400, Chicago, Ill. 60603. *Tel:* (312) 346-3458. Eugene J. McClory, Pres.

PURPOSE. A library and publisher providing training in principles and methods of Adlerian psychology. *Specialization:* principles and techniques of Adlerian psychology.
PUBLICATIONS. Books on teachings of Alfred Adler, role playing, transactional analysis, discipline, counseling, family life, classroom dynamics. Films, videotapes, sound recordings, bibliographies, and indexes on similar topics. Student guidebooks, monographs, back issues of journals also offered. Payment required with order.

G6. ALLYN AND BACON, INC., College Division, Rockleigh, N.J. 07647.*

PURPOSE. A publisher of college, junior college, and professional texts. *Specialization*: textbooks.
PUBLICATIONS. Three-hundred page catalog lists books in such categories as biology, biochemistry, organic chemistry, plus psychology (developmental, educational, statistics). Series on physical activity and on sports education for physical education; another series is on social psychology. Detailed descriptions of texts in catalog, along with outlines of contents. Payment not required with orders from bookstores; required with individual order.

G7. AMERICAN JOURNAL OF EPIDEMIOLOGY, School of Hygiene and Public Health, Johns Hopkins University, 615 N. Wolfe St., Baltimore, Md. 21205. *Tel:* (301) 955-3441. Frances Stark, Tech. Ed.

PURPOSE. To publish original field and laboratory studies on the occurrence and distribution of endemic and epidemic diseases with articles on infectious and noninfectious acute and chronic diseases and statistical methodology. Reviews and Commentary section contains signed editorials and reviews of various aspects of epidemiologic research. *Specialization:* epidemiology.
SPECIAL INFORMATION SERVICES. Mailing list is for sale.
PUBLICATION. Journal, the *American Journal of Epidemiology* (monthly) subscription $40/yr. in U.S.; $10 for public health students.
INQUIRY ADDRESS. E. A. Delcher, Bus. Mgr., American Journal of Epidemiology, 615 N. Wolfe St., Baltimore, Md. 21205. *Tel:* (301) 955-3441.

G8. THE AMERICAN JOURNAL OF NURSING COMPANY, Educational Services Division, 10 Columbus Circle, New York, N.Y. 10019. *Tel:* (212) 582-8820. Philip E. Day, R.N., Publishing Dir.

PURPOSE. To publish nursing periodicals and print and audiovisual educational materials. *Specialization:* nursing.
PUBLICATIONS. *American Journal of Nursing, Nursing Outlook, Nursing Research, International Nursing Index, MCN—the American Journal of Maternal Child Nursing.* Thirty-two-page catalog of reprints, supplements, programmed instruction, films, filmstrips, slides, audiocassettes, syllabi, and videotapes. Payment required with order under $10.

G9. AMERICAN PRINTING HOUSE FOR THE BLIND, INC., 1839 Frankfort Ave., Box 6085, Louisville, Ky. 40206. Finis E. Davis, Vice-Pres. and Gen. Mgr.

PURPOSE. Publication of books and music scores for the blind. *Specialization:* publications for the blind.
PUBLICATIONS. Hundreds of titles in all subjects. Extensive catalogs. Braille, large type, talking books, and materials for note-taking and transcribing. Health materials aimed at school-age audiences: personal health, hygiene, biology, psychology texts. Payment required with order.

G10. AMS PRESS, 56 E. 13 St., New York, N.Y. 10003.*

PURPOSE. To publish reprint editions of monographs and series. *Specialization:* reprints.
PUBLICATIONS. Many in social sciences, but some in history of medicine. Their *History of Medicine* catalog lists 90 monographs in reprint. Most are histories of medicine and not copies of primary sources. Prices are between $10 and $30. The *Clio Medica* series of 22 volumes is a set of primers on the history of medicine.

G11. ARCO PUBLISHING COMPANY, INC., 219 Park Ave. S., New York, N.Y. 10003. *Tel:* (212) 573-6600. Milton Gladstone, Pres.

PURPOSE. To publish a variety of books in the test-preparation field and books in health and medicine. *Specialization:* publishing of books in all fields.
PUBLICATIONS. Free catalog lists approximately 110 books on health, medicine, and fitness for the layman. Review series on nursing, anatomy, physiology, and other topics using multiple-choice questions to self-examine. Majority of books concern nutrition, how to live longer, and advocacy of various vitamins or diets. Payment required with order under $25.

G12. BALLINGER PUBLISHING COMPANY, 17 Dunster St., Harvard Square, Cambridge, Mass. 02138.*

PURPOSE. To publish books on public policy, government, ecology, health, education, and other fields. *Specialization:* public affairs, economics, and public health.
PUBLICATIONS. 112-page catalog includes selections in population and demography, health policy and health administration (topics such as *The Diffusion of Medical Technology, Assuring Quality in Medical Care, Equity in Health Services, Writer's Guide to Medical Journals*), alcoholic and drug abuse (*The Persistent Poppy, Alcohol and Alcohol Problems*), psychiatry, psychology, and mental health (*Geropsychology, The Regulation of Encounter Groups*), and other concerns. Payment required with order under $10.

G13. BARTEL DENTAL BOOK COMPANY, INC., 112 Crown St., Brooklyn, N.Y. 11225. *Tel:* (212) 772-8170. Thelma Loeb, Pres.

PURPOSE. A dealer in mail-order out-of-print books and periodicals, covering dentistry and allied fields. *Specialization:* out-of-print dental publications.
PUBLICATIONS. Bartel publishes one book on myofunctional therapy (diagnosis and treatment of abnormal swallowing habits). Accompanied by motivational tape for patient backed by taped discussion for practitioner, $30. Also set of five tapes on myofunctional therapy to expand on text, $60/tape. Payment required with order.

G14. BASIC BOOKS, INC., 10 E. 53 St., New York, N.Y. 10022.*

PURPOSE. To publish books in social sciences, psychology, and psychiatry. *Specialization:* social science, psychology, and psychiatry.
PUBLICATIONS. Recent releases include *Interpretation of Schizophrenia; Perception and Understanding in Young Children; Advice and Dissent: Scientists in the Political Arena;* the classic by Claude Levi-Strauss, *Structural Anthropology; An Introduction to the Philosophy of Science; The Discovery of the Unconscious: The History and Evaluation of Dynamic Psychiatry;* plus a history of psychology, and report on drug companies' collusion in suppressing information during thalidomide scare of several years ago— "the triumph of marketing skill over conscience" (*Thalidomide and the Power of the Drug Companies*). Catalogs available. Payment not required with order.

G15. BIO MONITORING APPLICATIONS, INC., 270 Madison Ave., New York, N.Y. 10016.* *Tel:* (212) 258-2724.

PURPOSE. A producer of information on yoga, biofeedback, and relaxation techniques. *Specialization:* biofeedback and self-control.

PUBLICATIONS. Books, tapes, and journals; self-control, autogenic therapy, muscle-relaxation training, and other related topics. Journal *Biofeedback and Self Control* (four issues), $15 for individuals.

G16. BOSTON UNIVERSITY MEDICAL CENTER, Office of Postgraduate Education, 720 Harrison Ave., Suite 206, Boston, Mass. 02118. *Tel:* (617) 247-1973. R. H. Egdahl, M.D., Dir.

PURPOSE. A medical center composed of Medical School, Dental School, Graduate Dental School, University Hospital, and affiliated teaching hospitals. *Specialization:* medical education.
PUBLICATIONS. Books published through Publishing Sciences Group in Acton, Mass., are manuscripts of Boston University's postgraduate education programs. Publications currently being prepared include titles of hypertension, diagnostic oncologic radiology, and nutrition in the practice of medicine. Payment not required with order.

G17. R. R. BOWKER COMPANY, 1180 Ave. of the Americas, New York, N.Y. 10036. Robert Asleson, Pres.

PURPOSE. To publish bibliographic material covering all media. Selection includes guides to publishing industry, librarianship, and multimedia programs. *Specialization:* bibliographic guides.
PUBLICATIONS. 110 page-book list plus flyers on new publications. Of health interest are bibliography on *Sex and Sex Education*, bibliographies of medical professional societies and their publications. Dieters can find information on special cookbooks and pamphlets in *The Diet Food Finder*. Multimedia resources include *Educational Media Yearbook* (ed. James M. Brown), with Multimedia Resources Directory contained in it, listing suppliers of health and medical materials, among others. *Multimedia Materials for Afro-American Studies* emphasizes films, lists documentaries of particular interest to black students, including medical care and sex education in topics considered. Large selection in librarianship includes guidebooks advising on setting up multimedia collections, touches on health, medicine, psychology, and related fields. Many guides to serials both in- and out-of-print, covering medical journals and scientific publications. International directory of *Irregular Serials and Annuals*. Comprehensive book list with detailed descriptions. Payment not required with order.

BRAIN INFORMATION SERVICE *See* E5

G18. BRUNNER/MAZEL, INC., 64 University Place, New York, N.Y. 10003.*

PURPOSE. To publish books in psychiatry, psychoanalysis, psychology, and child development. *Specialization:* books in behavioral sciences.
PUBLICATIONS. Books are aimed at mental health professionals, hospitals, libraries, and others in the behavioral sciences. Group therapy, adolescence, *World History of Psychiatry*, mental retardation, minimal brain dysfunction; several selections on use of drawings in diagnosis, as well as on more traditional Rorschach test. Racism, social conditioning, cognition, and other areas are also included. Payment not required with institutional order.

G19. BURGESS PUBLISHING COMPANY, 7108 Ohms Lane, Minneapolis, Minn. 55435* *Tel:* (612) 831-1344.

PURPOSE. To produce instructional books and film loops. *Specialization:* books.
PUBLICATIONS. Books on physical education, physical therapy, educational psychology, first aid, self-destructive behavior, hospital dietetics, nursing, pharmacy, pharmacology, biological sciences, and microbiology; super-8 film loops in biology. Payment not required with order.

G20. BUTTERWORTHS PROFESSIONAL AND EDUCATIONAL PUBLISHERS, 161 Ash St., Reading, Mass. 01867.

PURPOSE.To publish texts and scientific books. *Specialization:* books in medicine.
PUBLICATIONS. Large and varied selection in all areas of medicine, described in separate folders for ob/gyn, internal medicine, pediatrics, pathology, cardiology, surgery, and other fields. Also separate list of medical books by author. Payment not required with order.

G21. CAMBRIDGE UNIVERSITY PRESS, 32 E. 57 St., New York, N.Y. 10022. *Tel:* (212) 688-8888. Jack Schulman, Dir.

PURPOSE. To publish and distribute scholarly publications of Cambridge University Press in the United States. *Specialization:* scholarly publications.
PUBLICATIONS. Impressive volumes in biology, physiology, psychology, and medicine. New books on biology include ones on animal cytology, fetal and neofetal physiology, excitable cells, and others. Medical texts and monographs. Journals on hygiene, biological reviews, cell science, embryology, and parasitology. Payment required with order; Master Charge or BankAmericard accepted.

G22. CORNELL UNIVERSITY PRESS, 104 Roberts Place, Ithaca, N.Y. 14850. *Tel:* (607) 273-5155. Roger Howley, University Publisher and Dir.

PURPOSE. The book-publishing division of Cornell University, publishing general and specialized nonfiction in all fields. *Specialization:* scholarly publishing.
PUBLICATIONS. Fifty-five-page Complete Catalog. Medical titles concern public health and history of medicine. Also selections in veterinary medicine. Payment required with individual order.

G23. CRC PRESS, INC., 18901 Cranwood Parkway, Cleveland, Ohio 44128. *Tel:* 475-9000. B. J. Starkoff, Pres.

PURPOSE. To publish reference books and journals serving medical and scientific communities. *Specialization:* medicine and science.
PUBLICATIONS. Books and periodicals; reference books, handbooks, and journals. Most well known is CRC *Handbook of Chemistry and Physics.* Payment not required with order.

G24. F. A. DAVIS COMPANY/PUBLISHERS, 1915 Arch St., Philadelphia, Pa. 19103.*

PURPOSE. To publish textbooks, reference books, and slide sets in the fields of medicine, nursing, and the life and behavioral sciences. *Specialization:* medicine.

PUBLICATIONS. The spring 1975 catalog lists nearly 200 in-print titles covering most areas of medicine and nursing. The audiovisuals are slides with printed manuals and sometimes accompanying audiotapes. All titles are high quality. The average price per volume is $20. Payment not required with order.

G25. JOHN DAY, ABELARD-SCHUMAN, 666 Fifth Ave., New York, N.Y. 10019. *Tel:* (212) 489-2200. Lewis Gillenson, Pres.

PUBLICATIONS. Eighty-page catalog of Thomas Y. Crowell trade books; 29-page catalog of Abelard-Schuman, Criterion, and Windmill Books, including general medical (in area of health for general audiences), natural science, and some biology and psychology. Forty-five-page John Day Company catalog includes some general medical and public health books.

G26. DENEDCO OF DALLAS, Box 12597, Dallas, Tex. 75225. Lucille L. Bell, Mgr.

PURPOSE. To publish books. *Specialization:* dentistry.

PUBLICATIONS. Dental textbook by Welden E. Bell, D.D.S., clinical professor of oral surgery, University of Texas Southwestern Medical School of Dallas. Book entitled *Orofacial Pains—Differential Diagnosis*, 1973. Payment not required with order. If order prepaid, publisher prepays postage. Book is available with usual library and dealer discounts from distributor: J. A. Majors Medical Book Co., Box 47552, Dallas, Tex. 75247, or telephone Mr. W. H. Majors (214) 631-1470.

G27. DOVER PUBLICATIONS, INC., 180 Varick St., New York, N.Y. 10003. *Tel:* (212) 255-3755. Hayward Cirker, Pres.

PURPOSE. A book publisher specializing in paperback reprints. *Specialization:* paperback reprints in all fields.

PUBLICATIONS. Health sciences field covered by several books on psychology, history of medicine; good selection on biology. Free catalog gives detailed descriptions of all books. Payment required with order.

G28. DRUG INTELLIGENCE PUBLICATIONS, 1241 Broadway, Hamilton, Ill. 62341.* Donald E. Fraucke, Pres.

PURPOSE. To publish books and audiotapes on pharmacy for the pharmacist, physician, and nurse. *Specialization:* pharmacy.

PUBLICATIONS. About fifteen monograph titles, primarily on clinical pharmacy topics. Eight sets of audiotapes with reference manuals, prepared by the Extension Division in Pharmacy at the University of Wisconsin for continuing education are also available for purchase. Also, journal *Drug Intelligence and Clinical Pharmacy* (monthly), $18/yr. Payment not required with order. Billing charge $1 for order less than $30.

G29. EDUCATORS PROGRESS SERVICE, INC., Randolph, Wisc. 53956. R. H. Suttles, Publisher.

PURPOSE. To publish guides to sources of free audiovisual materials for use in classroom. *Specialization:* Free audiovisual materials.
PUBLICATIONS. Guides to free materials run to about 250 pages for each volume. Volumes cover *Guidance Materials*; *Science*; *Free Tapes, Scripts and Transcriptions*; *Health, Physical Education and Recreation.* Hefty guides advise user as to sources, contents of available materials, restrictions on use, whether or not item can be kept. Editions of each volume updated regularly to insure currency, and each has separate index on availability of items for Australians and Canadians. Films, filmstrips, slides, overhead projections, audio- and videotapes, scripts (of speeches, etc.), phono discs, bulletins, pamphlets, charts, exhibits, posters, maps, magazines, and books—some 2500 free items per volume. In *Health* catalog, listings include hygiene, safety, careers in health, first aid, nutrition, sex, fitness. In *Science,* items in biology and ecology among listings, and *Guidance* covers careers in health (along with advice to girls on how to be charming). Tapes catalog lists acupuncture, hyperactive children, mental health and diet among topics on tapes and discs. Note: films are from varied sources, from government agencies and the U.S. Army to National Bowling Council and McDonnell-Douglas Aircraft Corp. Industrial films may have to be considered in terms of public relations content as well as topics. Any charges (shipping, insurance) are specified by agency handling particular item listed.

G30. ELSEVIER/EXCERPTA MEDICA/NORTH HOLLAND, 52 Vanderbilt Ave., New York, N.Y. 10017. *Tel:* (212) MU 6-5277. J. J. Kels, Pres.

PURPOSE. To publish upper level scientific and technical books and journals. *Specialization:* scholarly publications.
PUBLICATIONS. Monthly listings or new books; 200-page complete catalog covering medicine, biology, earth sciences, social sciences, physical sciences, and economics. Many journals carried. Payment in Dutch florins not required with order.

ENVIRONMENT INFORMATION CENTER, INC. *See* E14

G31. EXCERPTA MEDICA B. V., Keizersgracht 305, Amsterdam, Netherlands. J. van Manen, Dir.

PURPOSE. To publish medical information for professionals in books, audiovisuals, and computer tapes. *Specialization:* medical publishing.
SPECIAL INFORMATION SERVICES. Computer and translation services.
PUBLICATIONS. Audiovisual patient counseling for chronic diseases, medical translation service, monographs, current and retrospective abstracts, newsletters, and computerized abstracts of 3,500 biomedical journals. Films for postgraduate medical education and audio- and videotapes. Wide-ranging services described in booklets. Payment required with order.

G32. FUTURA PUBLISHING COMPANY, 295 Main St., Box 298, Mount Kisco, N.Y. 10549.*

PURPOSE. To publish monographs and serials for professionals. *Specialization:* professional literature.
PUBLICATIONS. Catalog of books in medicine and allied health lists about 50

volumes, many of which are serial titles of a monographic nature. Most are specialty titles, but a few would appeal to more general audiences.

G33. GALE RESEARCH CO., Book Tower, Detroit, Mich. 48226.*

PURPOSE. To publish reference books and professional tools for the librarian. *Specialization:* reference books.
PUBLICATIONS. Several hundred books. Only seven are listed under the category "medicine" and are on subjects like *Folklore of the Teeth* and *The Quacks of Old London.* A number of other titles are of peripheral interest: *Encyclopedia of Associations, Statistics Sources, Research Centers Directory,* and a number of reprinted monographs. All books available on 30-day approval. Payment not required with order.

G34. HARPER AND ROW PUBLISHERS, INC., 10 E. 53 St., New York, N.Y. 10022. *Tel:* (212) 593-7000. Winthrop Knowlton, Pres.

PURPOSE. To publish print and media in wide area of subjects, including health and medicine. *Specialization:* publishing.
SPECIAL INFORMATION SERVICES. Loose-leaf update service in various medical specialties.
PUBLICATIONS. Catalogs in pure and applied sciences (college textbooks and audiovisual materials in biology, organic chemistry, nursing), health and education (psychology, mental health, motor learning, personal health); audiovisual materials (films, loops, slides, tapes on anatomy, physiology, biology, lab techniques, genetics and biochemistry, organic chemistry, human sexuality, nursing and allied health, speech disorders); multimedia program "The Nursing Process" contains 11 training units for use by nursing schools and training hospitals, includes micrograph 35mm slides, films on hematology, urinalysis, and parasitology. Catalog of medical publications runs 60 pages, and includes mostly monographs on all areas of internal medicine and lab techniques and practices. Also journals of *Pathology, Obstetrics-Gynecology, Ob-Gyn and Neonatal Nursing,* and *Clinical Ob and Gyn.* Payment not required with order.
INQUIRY ADDRESS: Medical Department, 2350 Virginia Ave., Hagerstown, Md. 21740. *Tel:* (301) 733-2700.

G35. HARVARD UNIVERSITY PRESS, 79 Garden St., Cambridge, Mass. 02138. *Tel:* (617) 495-2600. Arthur J. Rosenthal, Dir.

PURPOSE. To publish scholarly books and reference materials. *Specialization:* scholarly publishing.
PUBLICATIONS. 135-page catalog of books in print. Hundreds of titles, including, in Medicine and Public Health, internal medicine, surgery, immunology, and all areas of medicine. Community health plans, socialized medicine, training of health personnel; several volumes on health services and particular diseases as they occur in Massachusetts. Sociology of health-care delivery. Also tracts in biology, psychology, and psychiatry. Slides and audiotapes. Payment not required with order.

G36. HEALTH AFFAIRS PRESS, Box 425, Davis, Calif. 95616. *Tel:* (916) 758-1950. A. W. Schoen, Publisher.

PURPOSE. To publish books for general readers on health maintenance subjects. *Specialization:* health maintenance, preservation, and conservation.

G37. HILTZ AND HAYES PUBLISHING COMPANY, INC., 6304 Hamilton Ave., Cincinnati, Ohio 45224.*

PURPOSE. To provide multimedia programs on sex education, abortion, and marriage. *Specialization:* sex education, marriage, and abortion.
SPECIAL INFORMATION SERVICES. *Languages:* English, Spanish, and French.
PUBLICATIONS. Books, pamphlets, slides, audiocassettes, filmstrips, and records. Approach taken is pro-life, noncondemnatory.

G38. HOLDEN-DAY, INC., 500 Sansome St., San Francisco, Calif. 94111. *Tel:* (415) 433-0220. Frederick H. Murphy, Pres.

PURPOSE. To publish college texts. *Specialization:* college texts.
PUBLICATIONS. Introductory readings in community psychology and community mental health; *Introductory Biochemistry*; *Molecular Basis of Mutation*; *Immunogenetics*; *Chemical Modification of Proteins*.

G39. HUMAN SCIENCES PRESS, 72 Fifth Ave., New York, N.Y. 10011.* *Tel:* (800) 257-0300; in New Jersey (800) 322-8150.

PURPOSE. To publish monographs and journals in sociology, education, psychology, health, and related fields. *Specialization:* books and journals in behavioral and social sciences.
PUBLICATIONS. Listed in 40-page catalog. Books cover several topics in area of child study, notably child psychiatry and psychology, child care, development and rearing. Also treated are community mental health, day care and early education, higher education, health-care delivery, psychotherapy, general psychology, school psychology. Varied selection in sex, marriage, and the family, with special section on SIECUS (Sex Information and Education Council of the U.S.) publications: study guides on various fields of sex education and sexual behavior, bibliographies in sex education for mentally retarded, reports on status of sex research, series on "The Professional as Sex Educator" (for social workers, guidance counselors, et al.). Section on "Thanatology" (suicide, social aspects of death). *Community Mental Health Journal* (quarterly), $9.95/yr., introductory rate; *Journal of Community Health* (quarterly), $9.95/yr. introductory rate; and many other periodicals on child care, public health, and psychology, plus *Suicide* (quarterly). Payment not required with order.

INFORMATION CENTER FOR HEARING, SPEECH, AND DISORDERS OF HUMAN COMMUNICATION *See* E21

G40. JASON ARONSON, INC., Book Publishers, 59 Fourth Ave., New York, N.Y. 10003.* *Tel:* (212) 677-1280. Jason Aronson, M.D., Chief Executive Officer.

PURPOSE. To publish books and audiotapes in behavioral sciences and social sciences for mental health professionals. *Specialization:* behavioral and social sciences.
PUBLICATIONS. Books and tapes described in 184-page catalog, $1. Detailed run-

downs on available volumes, illustrated with interesting "experimental" photos. Subjects covered include child-adolescent psychology, therapy, analysis, social psychology, group therapy and encounter, pastoral counseling, crime and delinquency; series of 12 volumes on "Classical Analysis and Its Applications." Large tape cassette collection, concentrating on psychoanalysis and psychotherapy; also dealing with adolescence, day care, paranoia, self-actualization, and other fields of behavior. *Psychotherapy and Social Science Review* (monthly) available to mental health professionals in three editions: Regular, Psychoanalysts', and Pastors'. *Review* is guide to newly published works in fields of psychology and social science, sent to members of Psychotherapy and Social Science Book Club run by Jason Aronson, Inc. Payment not required with order.

G41. JOHNS HOPKINS UNIVERSITY PRESS, Charles and 34 St., Baltimore, Md. 21218. *Tel:* (301) 366-9600. Jack Goellner, Dir.

PURPOSE. To publish scholarly books and journals.

PUBLICATIONS. Selections large and varied. Books currently in print include volumes on environment, genetics, history of medicine, medical sciences, psychiatry, psychology, and public health. Of interest is recent addition of translation of K. L. Kahlbaum's *Catatonia*. Medical journals are *Bulletin of the History of Medicine* and *The Johns Hopkins Medical Journal*. Series on International Health features five monographs on health problems in Third World countries. Net payment due 30 days after receipt of book.

G42. JOHNSON ASSOCIATES, INC., Box 1017, Greenwich, Conn. 06830.* *Tel:* (203) 661-7602.

PURPOSE. To produce for archival purposes on silver halide film scholarly periodicals in microfiche format. Purchasers must be subscribers to paper editions. Volumes may be ordered individually.

PUBLICATIONS. About 500 periodical titles in microfiche. All are available from volume 1 on. About 20 percent are in health areas as of the end of 1975. In addition, a collection of original nonpublished selected psychology documents, entitled JSAS, and the monographic series *Archives of Psychology* are also available. A catalog of these publications is available. Payment not required with order.

G43. LANGE MEDICAL PUBLICATIONS, Drawer L, 795 Altos Oaks Dr., Los Altos, Calif. 94022. *Tel:* (415) 948-4526. Donald Peglow, Comptroller.

PURPOSE. To publish medical textbooks for medical students. *Specialization:* medicine.

SPECIAL INFORMATION SERVICES. *Languages:* English, Spanish, Italian, Portuguese, Polish, Turkish, Japanese, Greek, Serbo-Croatian, German, French, Czech, Vietnamese, Dutch, Romanian, and Hindi.

PUBLICATIONS. Small selection of current medical books cover ob/gyn, poisoning, clinical ECGs, microbiology, and other areas. Impressive number of foreign-language translations of current listings. Payment required with order unless credit established.

G44. LEA & FEBIGER, 600 Washington Sq., Philadelphia, Pa. 19106. *Tel:* (215) 922-1330. Christian C. Febiger Spahr, Sr., Senior Partner.

PURPOSE. A publisher. *Specialization:* books in life sciences.
PUBLICATIONS. Eighty-page catalog of books in life sciences. Texts, monographs, and handbooks in anatomy, dentistry, genetics, technology, labs, podiatry, preventive medicine, and veterinary medicine, all areas of medicine and health. Series on ob-gyn. Fourteen days approval. Payment not required with order.

G45. LEARNING DYNAMICS, INC., 167 Corey Rd., Boston, Mass. 02146.*

PURPOSE. An educational publishing company. *Specialization:* behaviors.
PUBLICATIONS. Multimedia programs include audiocassettes combined with exercise books. Programs are concerned with human behavior sciences. Brochure describes, for example, dynamics of mood control. Two-week trial period offered. Prepayment advised.

G46. LEXINGTON BOOKS, D.C. Heath and Company, 125 Spring St., Lexington, Mass. 02173.*

PURPOSE. To publish books "designed primarily to provide advanced research to professional and academic individuals." *Specialization:* scholarly books.
PUBLICATIONS. A special, separate, health sciences catalog lists about 40 titles, primarily in health administration and economics. A standing order program is available to libraries. If payment accompanies order, buyer does not have to pay delivery charges.

G47. MEDICAL ECONOMICS COMPANY, 550 Kinderkamack Rd., Oradell, N.J. 07649. *Tel:* (201) 262-3030. Charles P. Daly, Pres.

PURPOSE. To publish magazines, journals, catalogs, compendia, cassettes, and specialized communications of help to health-care field. (Services generally restricted to subscribers and readers.) *Specialization:* publications for health professions.
PUBLICATIONS. Concentration in books and periodicals on business aspects of medical practice. *Medical Economics* magazine (fortnightly), *Hospital Physician* (monthly), *RN* for registered nurses, *Product Management* for drug and cosmetic industries, desk references for specialists. Manuals on medical problems encountered in practice, and those encountered on stock exchange. Guides (books and audiotape cassettes) on tax shelters, investments, portfolios, retirement, money management, testifying in court, malpractice situation, and bill collection. Also continuing education on tape cassettes. Some publications free (controlled circulation); for others, payment required with order.

G48. MEDICAL EXAMINATION PUBLISHING COMPANY, INC., 65-36 Fresh Meadow Lane, Flushing, N.Y. 11365. *Tel:* (212) 463-1052. David C. Dimendberg, Pres.

PURPOSE. To publish books in medical and allied health fields. *Specialization:* medical and allied health fields.
PUBLICATIONS. Sixty-page catalog of exam review books, self-assessment books,

texts, monographs, manuals in medicine, dentistry, nursing, and allied health professions. Largest selection in ob/gyn, pediatrics, psychiatry, and surgery. Also audiotapes. Payment not required with order.

G49. MICROCARD EDITIONS, Denver Technological Center, 5500 S. Valentia Way, Englewood, Colo. 80110. *Tel:* (303) 771-2600.

PURPOSE. To publish in microform periodical backfiles and subscriptions and collections of reports and books in microform.
PUBLICATIONS. About 800 periodical titles available in various formats. roughly 10 percent in the health field. Formats include microfilm and -fiche. Invoice accompanies shipment; all payment terms are 30 days net.

G50. MIT PRESS, 28 Carleton Street, Cambridge, Mass. 02142. *Tel:* (617) 253-5254. Frank Verbanowski, Dir.

PURPOSE. To publish scholarly books in sciences and other areas. *Specialization:* books. Payment required with orders under $10.

G51. THE C. V. MOSBY COMPANY, 11830 Westline Industrial Dr., St. Louis, Mo. 63141. *Tel:* (314) 872-8370. Robert Strain, Pres.

PURPOSE. To publish medical, dental, and nursing books and textbooks. *Specialization:* largest selection of medical books is in ophthalmology; in dental books, orthodontics and prosthetics; in medical-surgical nursing; and college-level biology and physical education.
SPECIAL INFORMATION SERVICES. *Languages:* Arabic, Dutch, Finnish, French, German, Greek, Italian, Japanese, Persian, Polish, Portuguese, Serbo-Croatian, Sinhala, Spanish, Thai, and Turkish.
PUBLICATIONS. Textbooks, professional guides, and journals for medical and dental professionals, college-level students, and professional and practical nurses. Free price list of over 600 references and texts, some of which come with View-Master stereoscopic slides. Also publishes nine medical journals: *American Heart Journal, American Journal of Obstetrics and Gynecology, Clinical Pharmacology and Therapeutics, Investigative Ophthalmology, Surgery,* and the journals of *Allergy and Clinical Immunology, Laboratory and Clinical Medicine, Pediatrics,* and *Thoracic and Cardiovascular Surgery.* Dental journals include *Oral Surgery, Oral Medicine, Oral Pathology, American Journal of Orthodontics,* and *Journal of Prosthetic Dentistry.* Nursing is covered by *Heart and Lung: The Journal of Critical Care.* Subscriptions available at institutional, personal, or student intern rates. Price list free; faculty members eligible for complimentary or approval copies.

G52. NATIONAL LEARNING CORPORATION, 20 DuPont St., Plainview, N.Y. 11803. *Tel:* (516) 935-5800.

PURPOSE. To publish study guides for standardized exams. *Specialization:* "prep" books for those taking standardized examinations for government service and higher education.
PUBLICATIONS. Free catalog lists several hundred study guides, most prices $6-$7.50. Largest selection are for civil service exams; also available are guides for

teacher's license, Graduate Record, and regents' external degree exams. Of interest in health sciences field are those books covering exams for nurses, medical school admission, and health professionals entering the civil service. Payment required with order.

NATIONAL TECHNICAL INFORMATION SERVICE *See* E28

G53. NOYES DATA CORPORATION, Mill Rd. at Grand Ave., Park Ridge, N.J. 07656.* *Tel:* (201) 391-8484.

PURPOSE. To publish technical and business books in hard cover.
PUBLICATIONS. Catalog lists technical books in areas which include food, the environment, chemistry, pharmaceuticals, and energy. Publisher claims its binding method allows faster publication and therefore up-to-date information. If payment prepaid, postage does not have to be included.

G54. PRENTICE-HALL, Englewood Cliffs, N.J. 07632.*

PURPOSE. To publish textbooks and produce film loops. *Specialization:* textbooks and film loops.
PUBLICATIONS. 360-page catalog of materials. Series of 151 film loops on nursing skills and techniques for lectures or self-study. Book series on "Scientific Foundations of Nursing Practice." Reston Division's books, included in catalog, cover respiratory technology and dental hygiene. Payment not required with order.

G55. PRINCETON MICROFILM CORPORATION, Alexander Rd., Princeton, N.J. 08540.* *Tel:* (609) 452-2066.

PURPOSE. To publish scholarly research journals for libraries in 16mm or 35mm microfilm. *Specialization:* scholarly journals in microform.
PUBLICATIONS. The 1975/76 catalog includes approximately 2000 titles, about 400 of which are related to health. Many are foreign. Payment not required with order.

G56. PRINCETON UNIVERSITY PRESS, 41 William St., Princeton, N.J. 08540. *Tel:* (609) 452-4900. Herbert S. Bailey, Dir.

PURPOSE. To publish scholarly works. *Specialization:* scholarly publishing.
PUBLICATIONS. Catalogs for Spring 1975 and Fall 1974 additions, with separate catalogs for various fields covered by books in print. Princeton publishes Bollingen series of original contributions to scholarship, supported by Bollingen Foundation. Works in medicine are mainly concerned with its history. Payment required with orders not from persons with academic affiliation.
INQUIRY ADDRESS. Holly Danley, Princeton University Press, 41 William St., Princeton, N.J. 08540. *Tel:* (609) 452-4965.

G57. QUINTESSENCE PUBLISHING COMPANY, INC., 10 S. La Salle St., Chicago, Ill. 60603.*

PURPOSE. To publish a journal and a series of books in dentistry. *Specialization:* dentistry.

SPECIAL INFORMATION SERVICES. *Languages:* English, German, and Spanish.
PUBLICATIONS. The journal, *Quintessence International/ Dental Digest, the Journal of Practical Dentistry* is the English version of *Die Quintessenz,* $20/yr. The book series includes 18 titles on oral surgery, prosthodontics, practice management, pain, and others. They average about $50 each. All are scholarly. Payment not required with order.

G58. RESEARCH PRESS, Box 31779, Champaign, Ill. 61820.*

PURPOSE. To publish books and educational films.
PUBLICATIONS. Films include one on Skinner and one on family therapy. Books are geared toward educators and mental health specialists. They include titles on sexual and marital adjustment, autism, toilet training, mental retardation, and others. Most are paperbacks around $5, and less if ordered in quantity. Orders under $10 must be accompanied with payment. Prepaid orders receive priority. Established customers may be billed for orders over $10.

G59. ROUTLEDGE AND KEGAN PAUL, 9 Park St., Boston, Mass. 02108.* *Tel:* (617) 742-5863.

PURPOSE. A general publisher. *Specialization:* general audience books.
PUBLICATIONS. Books include some on alcoholism, family life, child abuse, mental illness, *Going to See the Doctor,* but most are on education, sociology, or history on a scholarly level.

G60. ST. MARTIN'S PRESS, 175 Fifth Ave., New York, N.Y. 10010.*

PURPOSE. To publish general interest monographs. *Specialization:* general interest books.
PUBLICATIONS. Most books are nonfiction of a scholarly nature. Those dealing with health include titles on weight reduction, childbirth, nutrition, addiction, *Living With Your Emphysema and Bronchitis,* and *Living With Your Ulcer.*

G61. SCHENKMAN PUBLISHING COMPANY, INC., 3 Mt. Auburn Place, Cambridge, Mass. 02138. *Tel:* (617) 492-4952. A. Schenkman, Pres.

PURPOSE. A book publisher. *Specialization:* social sciences.
PUBLICATIONS. Include *Socialization in Drug Abuse* and *Developments in the Field of Drug Abuse.* Payment not required with order.

G62. SCIENCE AND HEALTH PUBLICATIONS, 1740 N Street N.W., Washington, D.C. 20036.*

PURPOSE. To publish pooks and audiocassettes on science and health care. *Specialization:* health-care administration.
PUBLICATIONS. Books deal with hospital administration; health politics, law and administration; and audiocassettes on health policy and laws. Books are reasonably priced, many under $10, and cassettes are $8 or less. If prepaid, postage and handling will be covered.

G63. SIGNAL PRESS, National Women's Christian Temperance Union, 1730 Chicago Ave., Evanston, Ill. 60201.*

PURPOSE. To achieve prohibition of alcoholic drinks in the United States. *Specialization:* materials on alcohol and drugs.
PUBLICATIONS. Leaflets, booklets, books, and audiovisual materials on alcohol, tobacco, and other narcotics and their use, and hopefully their prohibition. Materials stress deleterious physical and social effects of Demon Rum, promote good citizenship. Coloring books, exhibits, posters. *The Union Signal* (monthly), $3/yr; *The Young Crusader* (monthly) aimed at under-12 readers. Payment required with order.

G64. SIMON AND SCHUSTER, 630 Fifth Ave., New York, N.Y. *Tel:* (212) CI 5-6400. Leon Samkin, Chmn. of the Board.

PURPOSE. A general-interest publisher. *Specialization:* book publishing.
PUBLICATIONS. Fiction and nonfiction, cloth and paperbacks. Health books appeal to general audience, concern personal fitness, nutrition, sex, and psychotherapy. Payment required with individual order.

G65. CHARLES B. SLACK, INC., 6900 Grove Rd., Thorofare, N.J. 08086. *Tel:* (609) 848-1000. Charles B. Slack, Pres.

PURPOSE. To publish medical journals and textbooks. (Services restricted to professional medical, health, and safety groups.) *Specialization:* health-care publications.
PUBLICATIONS. Books and periodicals in all areas of health care, primary emphasis on nursing. National office for American Federation for Clinical Research, American Society of Nephrology, American Gastroenterological Association, American Society of Hematology. Advertising representative for numerous medical journals, offers convention and exhibit management services for professional medical, health, and fire safety organizations. Payment not required with order.

G66. SPECIAL CHILD PUBLICATIONS, 4535 Union Bay Place N.E., Seattle, Wash. 98105.* *Tel:* (206) 522-2036.

PURPOSE. To publish books for educators dealing with special children. *Specialization:* special education.
PUBLICATIONS. Books include titles concerned with auditory and sight problems as well as general educational methods, learning theory, and behavior. Most are available in reasonably priced paperback editions. Payment required with individual order. Purchaser must also pay shipping and handling fees.

G67. SPECTRUM PUBLICATIONS, INC., 86-19 Sancho St., Holliswood, N.Y. 11423. *Tel:* (212) 479-9360. Maurice Ancharoff, Pres.

PURPOSE. To publish information on medicine, biology, biochemistry, psychiatry/psychology, health-care delivery, and other subjects for a professional and student audience. *Specialization:* biology, medicine, psychiatry/psychology, medical sociology, and health-care management.
PUBLICATIONS. *Addictive Diseases* (quarterly), journal audiotape series on psycho-

pharmacology; also books and slides. Price lists available. Payment not required with order.

G68. SPRINGER PUBLISHING COMPANY, 200 Park Ave. S., New York, N.Y. 10003. *Tel:* (212) 475-2494. Ursula Springer, Pres.

PURPOSE. To publish books for the health field, primarily nurses and paramedical personnel, but also medicine, veterinary medicine, and pharmacology. *Specialization:* medicine, nursing, public health, and pharmacology.
PUBLICATIONS. Thirty-five-page catalog of psychology, neurology, community mental health, and gerontology books for professionals and general readership. Nursing texts on problem-oriented nursing, management, research, cancer care, psychiatric care, and nursing dictionary. Medical catalog of 30 titles, covering urban health services, abortion, personality and aging, and psychiatry. Payment required with order under $10 or when opening new account.

G69. SPRINGER-VERLAG, Berlin, Federal Republic of Germany.* Axel Springer, Founder.

PURPOSE. Large West German publishing house, putting out books in both English and German.
PUBLICATIONS. English editions include definitive *Handbook of Sensory Physiology.* Eight volumes cover *Principles of Receptor Physiology* (Vol. I), *Chemical Senses* (Vol. IV), *Auditory Systems* (Vol. V), and *Perception* (Vol. VIII), among other aspects of receptor biology and biochemistry. Multidisciplinary treatment is intended as guide for graduate courses and seminars.

G70. STRATTON INTERCONTINENTAL MEDICAL BOOK CORPORATION, 381 Park Ave. S., New York, N.Y. 10016. *Tel:* (212) 683-5088. Dr. Henry M. Stratton, Pres.

PURPOSE. Publication of medical books and journals. U.S. distribution for selected foreign publishers. *Specialization:* books in medicine and psychology.
PUBLICATIONS. Largest selections in cardiology, gastroenterology, neurology, and psychology. Includes multivolume sets and monographs. Quarterly journal *Seminars in Thrombosis and Hemostasis,* $25/yr. in U.S.; *Israel Journal of Medical Sciences*; European medical journals in English. Payment not required with U.S. order.

G71. TAPLINGER PUBLISHING COMPANY, INC., 200 Park Ave. S., New York, N.Y . 10003. *Tel:* (212) 533-6110. Mrs. Terry Taplinger, Chief Executive Officer.

PURPOSE. Exclusive distributors in United States to bookstores and libraries of titles by Carnegie Endowment for International Peace, Garrett Publications, McKnight Publishing Company, and other presses. *Specialization:* psychology and parapsychology.
PUBLICATIONS. Some 18 titles in field of health and medicine listed in free catalog, including *Cookbook for Diabetics,* guides to childbirth, sexual health, and history of

medicine. McKnight books (distributed only to library and book trade) include *Introduction to Health Careers.* Payment required with order.

G72. TEACHERS COLLEGE PRESS, 1234 Amsterdam Ave., New York, N.Y. 10027. *Tel:* (212) 678-3927. Robert Bletter, Dir.

PURPOSE. To publish scholarly and instructive materials in field of education. Teachers College is part of Columbia University. *Specialization:* education.
PUBLICATIONS. Seventy-five-page catalog. Books include ones on child psychology in regard to education, childhood learning, behavior, education for the handicapped, growth and heredity, therapy, and cognition. Programmed instruction books in nursing education. *Teachers College Record* (quarterly), journal. Payment required with individual order.

G73. C. S. TEPFER PUBLISHING COMPANY, INC., Ridgefield, Conn. 06877.*
Charles Tepfer, Publisher.

PURPOSE. To publish guide to instructional videotapes. *Specialization:* information on obtaining educational videocassettes.
PUBLICATIONS. 130-page guide to over 4,100 programs on ¾" "U-Matic" videotape cassettes. Lists producers and distributors of titles, aimed at nonprofessional audiences. Health and safety, public health, and nursing. Payment not required with order.

G74. TRANSACTION INC., Rutgers University, New Brunswick, N.J. 08903.*

PURPOSE. To publish "scholarly, college and trade books of social science worth." *Specialization:* social science.
PUBLICATIONS. Books include several on environment, drugs, intelligence, social deviance, public health, and marriage. Prices are reasonable; most books under $10. Payment required with individual order; those from institutions over $10 can be billed.

G75. UNIPUB, Box 433, Murray Hill Station, New York, N.Y. 10016. *Tel:* (212) 686-4707. Wayne Kerwood, Pres.

PURPOSE. To distribute publications of United Nations agencies and other international organizations. Division of Xerox. *Specialization:* nutrition and nuclear medicine.
PUBLICATIONS. Price lists for publications of UN's International Atomic Energy Agency and the Food and Agriculture Organization contain descriptions of works available from those agencies via UNIPUB. UNIPUB also carries publications of other UN agencies. Of interest in health sciences field are FAO's books and manuals on personal nutrition, as well as nutritional problems facing the entire world. FAO also provides filmstrips that come with printed narration; periodicals; and commodity reports. IAEA's works cover radioisotopes in medicine, dosimetry, radiological safety, radiation biology, and radiopharmaceuticals. Reprints in nuclear medicine can be ordered as 35mm microfilm or bound xerographic copy. Payment required with order of $15 or less.

G76. UNIVERSITY OF CALIFORNIA PRESS, Berkeley, Calif. 94720.

PURPOSE. To publish scholarly books and journals. *Specialization:* scholarly publishing.
PUBLICATIONS. Catalog lists books in print 1974–1975, including about 40 titles in medicine, plus others in biology, and psychology. Much of medical literature is on history of medicine. Separate catalogs for new additions, Fall 1974 and Spring 1975. Payment not required with order.

G77. UNIVERSITY OF CHICAGO PRESS, 5801 Ellis Ave., Chicago, Ill. 60637. *Tel:* (312) 753-2594. Morris Philipson, Dir.

PURPOSE. To publish scholarly books, journals, and microfiche and offering limited-edition reprints of out-of-print books.
PUBLICATIONS. Catalogs issued periodically give complete rundowns on books added to the University of Chicago Press's extensive stock. Recent additions in health sciences include *Viruses Causing Common Respiratory Infections in Man* and *Health Care Politics: Ideological and Interest Group Barriers to Reform.* The press has produced a wide-ranging body of works in the health sciences, including notable texts in sociology and child development. Also available are six audiotape cassettes; these contain discussions by University of Chicago hospitals and clinics experts and are issued as the *University of Chicago Medical Reviews.* Topics covered include diabetes, hypertension, and hepatitis. Set of six tapes $45. Payment not required with order.
INQUIRY ADDRESS. Virginia Heiserman, Publicity Mgr., University of Chicago Press, 5801 Ellis Ave., Chicago, Ill. 60637. *Tel:* (312) 753-2595.

G78. UNIVERSITY OF ILLINOIS PRESS, 100 University Press Building, Urbana, Ill. 61801. *Tel:* (217) 333-0950. Miodrag Muntyan, Dir.

PURPOSE. To publish scholarly material. *Specialization:* scholarly publishing.
PUBLICATIONS. Books in special education, psychology, and rehabilitation, along with film on Illinois Psycholinguistic Abilities Test, which covers aphasia, manual communications, and childhood linguistics. Catalog of books in print in 1975 lists over 30 titles in medicine, and others in biology and psychology. Payment required with individual order.

G79. UNIVERSITY OF MINNESOTA PRESS, 2037 University Ave. S.E., Minneapolis, Minn. 55455.

PURPOSE. To publish scholarly books. *Specialization:* scholarly books.
PUBLICATIONS. Annotated book lists give titles in print. Selections on biology, psychiatry, and psychology, about 30 titles in medicine—for general and professional readership. Payment not required with order.

G80. UNIVERSITY OF MISSOURI PRESS, 107 Swallow Hall, University of Missouri, Columbia, Mo. 65201. *Tel:* 882-7641. Edward King, Dir.

PURPOSE. To publish scholarly books. *Specialization:* history, literature, and Missouriana.

PUBLICATIONS. Include some in medical sciences. Fall/Winter 1974 catalog includes bibliography of all books in print, and lists four in medical science. Payment required with individual order.

G81. UNIVERSITY OF PENNSYLVANIA PRESS, 3933 Walnut St., Philadelphia, Pa. 19104. *Tel:* (215) 243-6261. Robert Erwin, Dir.

PURPOSE. To publish scholarly materials. *Specialization:* books.
PUBLICATIONS. Biennial catalogs and complete list of publications. Some works in medicine, biology, and social aspects of health. Catalogs illustrated with "gallery" of photographs by one artist. Payment required with individual order.

G82. UNIVERSITY OF WISCONSIN PRESS, Box 1379, Madison, Wisc. 53701.* *Tel:* (608) 262-1116.

PURPOSE. To publish scholarly books and series.
PUBLICATIONS. Several hundred monographs and monographs in series include a number in the history of medicine, biology, health-care policy, public health nursing, medical bibliography, and biochemistry.

G83. UNIVERSITY PRESSES OF FLORIDA, 15 N.W. 15 St., Gainesville, Fla. 32603.*

PURPOSE. To publish scholarly books. *Specialization:* scholarly books.
PUBLICATIONS. About 300 volumes, some individual monographs and some in series. Of interest to health is the Center for Gerontology Studies and Programs, which has produced 23 volumes, including *Health Care Services for the Aged* and *Medical Care Under Social Security.* Payment not required with order.

G84. VANDERBILT UNIVERSITY PRESS, Box 1813, Station B, Nashville, Tenn. 37235. *Tel:* (615) 322-3585. Jane C. Tinsley, Office Mgr.

PURPOSE. To publish scholarly works. *Specialization:* humanities, social sciences, medicine, and regional.
PUBLICATIONS. Abraham Flexner Lectures cover autonomic transmitters, psychoanalysis, pediatrics, nutritional research, and a guide for the librarian in cataloging medical material, *Classification for Medical Literature.* Earlier studies in blood protein research, *Deafness in Childhood,* model therapeutic diets for health professionals, and a psychiatric appraisal of changing culture in New Guinea. Authoritative volume summarizing current knowledge of *Hemophilus Influenzae* (325 pages, $15), edited by Sarah H. W. Sell. *Diabetes and Pregnancy* is guide for prospective mothers with diabetes, 80 pages. Payment required with individual order.

G85. THE VIKING PRESS, 625 Madison Ave., New York, N.Y. 10022.*

PURPOSE. To publish general interest books in hard cover and paperback. Many are suitable for college use. *Specialization:* general interest books.
PUBLICATIONS. Catalogs list hundreds of monographs. None is strictly medicine, but many are in psychology. Some listed under science are on genetics and brain research. Educational discounts available if book is for class use.

G86. WAYNE STATE UNIVERSITY PRESS, Detroit, Mich. 48202.*

PURPOSE. To publish scholarly monographs. *Specialization:* scholarly books.
PUBLICATIONS. Several books are related to health and are about fertility, community mental health, exercise, first aid, and psychiatry. Examination copies are available if the book is under consideration and adopted as a class text. Short discounts given except for a few trade titles. Postage paid if remittance received with order.

G87. WESTERN PSYCHOLOGICAL SERVICES, 12031 Wilshire Blvd., Los Angeles, Calif. 90025.*

PURPOSE. To produce and distribute books, tests, materials, and journals to social scientists in psychology, education, medicine and rehabilitation. *Specialization:* psychology.
PUBLICATIONS. Catalog lists numerous tests and books on personality, intelligence, personnel, school readiness, counseling, retardation, reading, perceptual and motor skills, speech, delinquency, marriage, sex, medical forms, and aptitudes. *Human Behavior* is a monthly journal. Payment required with order.

G88. WILEY BIOMEDICAL DIVISION, John Wiley & Sons, 605 Third Ave., New York, N.Y. 10016. *Tel:* (212) 867-9800. Niels C. Buessem, Vice-Pres. and Gen. Mgr.

PURPOSE. To publish educational and reference material for total health-care market.
PUBLICATIONS. Books, films, slides, audiotapes, and periodicals in clinical medicine, basic medical sciences, nursing, and allied health fields. Payment not required with order.

G89. The WILLIAMS AND WILKINS COMPANY, 428 E. Preston St., Baltimore, Md. 21202. *Tel:* (301) 528-4000. Charles O. Reville, Jr., Pres.

PURPOSE. A publisher.
PUBLICATIONS. Books, films, slides, videotapes, and periodicals on medicine and allied sciences (nursing, veterinary medicine, pharmacy, and dentistry). Payment not required with order.

G90. THE H. W. WILSON COMPANY, 950 University Ave., Bronx, N.Y. 10452.*

PURPOSE. To publish indexes to current literature, reference tools, and professional literature for librarians. *Specialization:* library literature.
PUBLICATIONS. Indexes include *Readers Guide to Periodical Literature*, which covers general interest journals; *Vertical File Index*, which indexes general interest pamphlets; *Education Index*; *Library Literature*; and *Biological and Agricultural Index*, among others. These are useful tools for the non-professional layman or student looking for information on health. Prices for indexes are based on number of indexed periodicals a library receives and library budget.

G91. XEROX UNIVERSITY MICROFILMS, 300 N. Zeeb Rd., Ann Arbor, Mich. 48106.*

PURPOSE. University microfilms distributes dissertations, books, periodicals, and collections on microfilm or in photocopy form (on demand). *Specialization:* microform; dissertations.

PUBLICATIONS. Dissertation Abstracts International is the finding tool for dissertations which can then be ordered on film or photocopy from U. M. Several catalogs are available which list books available on demand. These are mostly out-of-print titles and the U. M. copies are considered reprints. One catalog is on medicine; microfilm copies of journals are available for an increasing number of medical titles. A flat fee is charged for each microfilm or photocopy, $4 and $10, respectively. Payment required with individual order.

G92. YEAR BOOK MEDICAL PUBLISHERS, INC., 35 E. Wacker Dr., Chicago, Ill. 60601. *Tel:* (312) 726-9733. W. F. Keller, Pres.

PURPOSE. To publish medical reference and textbooks and medical periodicals.

PUBLICATIONS. Fifty-page directory of publications. For professional audiences, including yearly compilations of abstracts from world's medical literature; all fields in medicine, psychiatry, and dentistry. Texts and monographs in many fields. Films, slides, and audiotapes. Payment not required with order.

H

Research Institutes

H1. CENTER FOR HEALTH ADMINISTRATION STUDIES, University of Chicago, 5720 S. Woodlawn Ave., Chicago, Ill. 60637.*

PURPOSE. To conduct program of research and education in social and economic aspects of medical care. Associated with Graduate Program in Hospital Administration and Graduate School of Business of the University of Chicago. *Specialization:* hospital management and health-care delivery

PUBLICATIONS. Listed in pamphlet. Bound volumes (available from publishers indicated in pamphlet) cover paying for medical care, community organization, health insurance, and other aspects of health-care delivery. Research reports, studies in hospital administration, special reports, lectures, symposia, and reprints are ordered directly from the center; deal with pertinent aspects of public health. Main concerns of materials are financial, administrative, and statistical, and are oriented toward management techniques involved in medical care, as might be expected from the center's affiliation with Chicago's Business School. Payment required with individual order; bulk orders for institutions can be arranged.

CARNATION RESEARCH LABORATORIES *See* F8

H2. CENTER OF ALCOHOL STUDIES, Rutgers University, New Brunswick, N.J. 08903. *Tel:* (201) 932-2190. John A. Carpenter, Dir.

PURPOSE. Research, education and training, documentation, and publications on alcohol use and abuse. *Specialization:* alcohol research, alcohol problems, drinking patterns, and alcohol education.

SPECIAL INFORMATION SERVICES. *Special collection:* collection of books and periodicals on alcohol and alcohol problems.

PUBLICATIONS. *Journal of Studies on Alcohol* (quarterly), with supplements. Books,

bibliographies, monographs, research data, pamphlets, and reprints. Reports on physiology, psychology, and treatment of alcoholism in society and industry. Payment required with order.
INQUIRY ADDRESS. Center of Alcohol Studies, Rutgers University, New Brunswick, N.J. 08903. *Tel:* (201) 932-3510.

H3. COLD SPRING HARBOR LABORATORY, Box 100, Cold Spring Harbor, N.Y. 11724. *Tel:* (516) 692-6660. James D. Watson, Dir.

PURPOSE. To do biological research. *Specialization:* biology and microbiology.
PUBLICATIONS. Abstracts subscriptions; course manuals used in lab's summer courses; results of symposia since 1941; much material on phages, RNA, DNA, cell culture, and genetics. Publications pamphlet available. Payment required with individual order.
INQUIRY ADDRESS. Publications Office, Cold Spring Harbor Laboratory, Box 100, Cold Spring Harbor, N.Y. 11724. *Tel:* (516) 692-6650, ext. 755.

H4. FELS RESEARCH INSTITUTE FOR THE STUDY OF HUMAN DEVELOPMENT—JENNIE MAY FELS MEMORIAL LIBRARY, 800 Livermore St., Yellow Springs, Ohio 45387. *Tel:* (513) 767-7324. Harriet Carter, Librarian.

PURPOSE. Library serves the needs of the parent organization, which is a nonprofit institution doing basic research in human development. *Specialization:* human development.
SPECIAL INFORMATION SERVICES. *Special collections:* growth genetics, pediatrics, social development, periodontology, motivated behavior, perceptual-cognitive development, as well as more commonly encountered medical fields.
PUBLICATIONS. Eighty-five-page catalog of publications. Lists 1,067 reprints of monographs and periodicals articles. Majority cover behavior, physiological aspects of psychology, psychomotor functions, child physiology, biochemistry, dental pathology, osteopathy, and comparative physiology as used in anthropology. Most subjects concern physical and psychological development of the child. Also pamphlets on purpose of the institute. Payment not required with order.

H5. THE FOX CHASE CANCER CENTER, 7701 Burholme Ave., Philadelphia, Pa. 19111. *Tel:* (215) 342-1000. Timothy R. Talbot, Jr., Pres.

PURPOSE. To do research into causes of and cures for cancer, care and rehabilitation for cancer patients, outreach programs in cancer control, and education for public and health professionals. *Specialization:* cancer research and treatment.
SPECIAL INFORMATION SERVICES. From January 1976, toll-free information and referral system for cancer patients and families, plus toll-free information and consultation system for health professionals.
PUBLICATIONS. Limited number of pamphlets and periodicals of primary interest to cancer patients and physicians specializing in cancer treatment. Attractive annual scientific reports.
INQUIRY ADDRESS. Information Service, Fox Chase Cancer Center, 7701 Burholme Ave., Philadelphia, Pa. 19111. *Tel:* (215) 342-1000.

H6. GRADUATE PROGRAM IN HOSPITAL AND HEALTH ADMINISTRA-
TION, University of Iowa, Iowa City, Iowa 52240. *Tel:* (319) 356-2593. Dr. Gerhard
Hartman, Chmn.

PURPOSE. To train future hospital and health administrators, planners, researchers,
and teachers.*Specialization:* hospitals and health care.
PUBLICATIONS. "Health Care Research" series of 20 titles on administration, cost
analyses, legislation, and medical education. Several concentrate on Iowa specifically. "Health Care Demonstration" series of eight titles on specific health-care
facilities. Payment required with order.

H7. INSTITUTE OF MEDICINE, National Academy of Sciences, 2101 Constitution Ave., N.W., Washington, D.C. 20418. *Tel:* (202) 389-6775. Donald S. Frederickson, M.D., Pres.

PURPOSE. A private institute dedicated to identifying problems and relationships
among segments of the health enterprise and to make recommendations to improve
quality of health care. *Specialization:* social and administrative aspects of nation's
health-care system.
PUBLICATIONS. Studies on costs of medical education, regulation of health industry,
HMO's, acute care, national health insurance, cancer programs, group bargaining by
health professionals, abortion, and medicine in China. Periodicals include annual
reports of institute and on federal health budget. Also bimonthly newsletter.

H8. NATIONAL CANCER CYTOLOGY CENTER, 150 Broad Hollow Rd.,
Melville, N.Y. 11746. *Tel:* (516) 427-0400. Ann L. Ayre, Exec. Dir.

PURPOSE. A nonprofit cancer research center. *Specialization:* cancer research.
PUBLICATIONS. Biannual journal, *Cancer Cytology,* covers immunology, pathology,
cancer diagnosis, and prevention and treatment, $6/yr. Educational pamphlets and
other material available on request. Payment required with subscription order.

H9. THE POPULATION COUNCIL, INC., 245 Park Ave., New York, N.Y. 10017.
Tel: (212) 687-8330. W. Parker Maulding, Acting Pres.

PURPOSE. To study problems created by increasing world population and relation of
population to material and cultural resources. *Specialization:* demography and
family planning for professional audiences.
SPECIAL INFORMATION SERVICES. *Languages:* French and Spanish.
PUBLICATIONS. Directed toward professional audience. *Studies in Family Planning*
(monthly); *Reports on Population/Family Planning* (6–8 issues/yr.); *Country
Profiles* (8–10 issues/yr.); bibliography with abstracts of important publications; *The
Population Chronicle* (quarterly), for decision makers who are not demographers.
French and Spanish versions of periodicals available. Council has biomedical
division and technical assistance and demographic divisions.

H10. PROSTHETIC-ORTHOTIC   CENTER—NORTHWESTERN   UNIVER-
SITY, 401 E. Ohio St., Chicago, Ill. 60611.*

PURPOSE. To rent and sell films on rehabilitation. *Specialization:* rehabilitation.
PUBLICATIONS. List of producer-distributors of films on prosthetics and orthotics.
Payment depends on particular distributor.

H11. REHABILITATION INSTITUTE OF CHICAGO, 401 E. Ohio St., Chicago,
Ill. 60611.*

PURPOSE. To rent and sell educational films. *Specialization:* films on rehabilitation.
PUBLICATIONS. Four films cover phenol nerve block, rehabilitation technique, and
paramedical career opportunities. Orders and inquiries should be directed to
attention of Photography Department. Payment not required with order.

H12. UNDERWRITERS LABORATORIES, INC., 207 E. Ohio St., Chicago, Ill.
60611. *Tel:* (312) 642-6969.

PURPOSE. A laboratory for testing products for public safety. *Specialization:* product
testing for safety.
SPECIAL INFORMATION SERVICES. Public Information and Education Service Department develops educational safety materials in all media.
PUBLICATIONS. Films on product testing by U.L., free for showings in schools.
Pamphlets on U.L.'s services, mobile home standards, vacuum cleaners, fire safety,
noise, annual report, career opportunities for engineers at U.L., lists of approved
products, 60 research bulletins. Public relations in public safety. Slides. Payment
required with order.

Source Index

ACI Films, Inc., B1

AIMS Instructional Media Services, Inc., B4

AMS Press, G10

AORN see Association of Operating Room Nurses, A105

AV-VID, Inc., B18

A-V Scientific Aids, B19

AVENS Audiovisual Education in Neurosurgery, B20

AVN see American Video Network

Abbot Laboratories, F1

Abelard-Schuman, Ltd. see John Day, Abelard-Schuman

Academic Press, Inc., G1

Academy of Psychosomatic Medicine, A1

Action on Smoking and Health, A2

Addison-Wesley Publishing Co., G2

Adler's Foreign Books, C1

Aero Medical Consultants, Inc., G3

Aeromedical Research Laboratory Library, D1

Aerospace Medical Association, A3

Aetna Life and Casualty, B2

Agency for Instructional Television, B3

Air Pollution Technical Information Center, E1

Akron City Health Dept., D2

Albany Medical College, B5

Albany Medical College—Union University, Schaffer Library of Health Sciences, E2

Albert Einstein College of Medicine, D. Samuel Gottesman Library, E3

Alcohol and Drug Problems Association of North America, A4

Aldine Publishing Co., G4

Alexander Graham Bell Association, A5

Alfred Adler Institute of Chicago, Inc., G5

Alfred Higgins Productions, B6

Allergy Foundation of America, A6

Allyn and Bacon, Inc., G6

Alternate Visions, Inc., B7

Alton Ochsner Medical Foundation, A7

American Academy of Allergy, A8

American Academy of Child Psychiatry, A9

American Academy of Dental Electrosurgery, A10

American Academy of Forensic Sciences, A11

American Academy of Health Administration, A12

American Academy of Ophthalmology and Otolaryngology, A13

American Academy of Optometry, A14

American Academy of Oral Pathology, A15

American Academy of Orthopaedic Surgeons, A16

American Academy of Osteopathy, A17

American Academy of Pediatrics, A18

American Association for Cancer Research, A19

American Association for Maternal and Child Health, A20

American Association for the Abolition of Involuntary Mental Hospitalization, A21

American Association for the Advancement of Science, A22

American Association of Bioanalysts, A24

American Association of Blood Banks, A25

American Association of Colleges of

Pharmacy, A26
American Association of Dental Schools, A27
American Association of Doctors' Nurses, A28
American Association of Foreign Medical Graduates, A29
American Association of Orthodontists, A30
American Association of Sex Educators and Counselors, A31
American Association for World Health, Inc., A23
American Association of Suicidology, A32
American Bar Association, A33
American Cancer Society, A34
American Chemical Society, A35
American Chiropractic Association, A36
American College Health Association, A37
American College of Cardiology Extended Learning, A38
American College of Nurse-Midwives, A39
American College of Radiology, A40
American College of Surgeons, A41
American College of Surgeons Surgical Film Library, A42
American Congress of Rehabilitation Medicine, A43
American Corrective Therapy Association, A44
American Council on Alcohol Problems, Inc., A45
American Dental Association, A46
American Dental Hygienists Association, A47
American Diabetes Association, A48
American Educational Films, B8
American Film Productions, Inc., B9
American Foundation for the Blind, A49
American Group Practice Association, A50
American Group Psychotherapy Association, A51
American Heart Association, A52
American Hospital Association, A53
American Institute of Physics, A54
American Institute of the History of Pharmacy, A55
American Journal of Epidemiology, G7
American Journal of Nursing Company, G8
American Library Association, A56
American Lung Association, A57
American Medical Association, A58
American Medical Record Association, A59
American Medical Student Association, A60
American Medical Technologists, A61

American Medical Women's Association, A62
American Natural Hygiene Society, A63
American Occupational Therapy Association, A64
American Optometric Association, A65
American Orthopsychiatric Association, A66
American Osteopathic Association, A67; see also American Academy of Osteopathy
American Pharmaceutical Association, A68
American Physical Therapy Association, A69
American Physiological Society, A70
American Podiatry Association, A71
American Printing House for the Blind, G9
American Professional Practice Association, A72
American Protestant Hospital Association, A73
American Psychiatric Association, A74
American Psychoanalytic Association, A75
American Psychological Association, A76
American Public Health Association, A77
American Schizophrenia Association see Huxley Institute
American School Health Association, A78
American Social Health Association, A79
American Society for Adolescent Psychiatry, A80
American Society for Clinical Pharmacology and Therapeutics, A81
American Society of Abdominal Surgeons, A87
American Society of Allied Health Professions, A88
American Society of Clinical Pathologists, A89
American Society for Gastrointestinal Endoscopy, A82
American Society of Hematology, A90
American Society of Hospital Attorneys, A91
American Society for Hospital Personnel Administration, A83
American Society of Hospital Pharmacists, A92
American Society of Internal Medicine, A93
American Society for Microbiology, A84
American Society for Pharmacology and Experimental Therapeutics, A85
American Society of Plastic and Reconstructive Surgeons see Educational Foundation of Plastic and Reconstructive Surgeons

American Society for Testing and Materials, A86

American Society of Tropical Medicine and Hygiene, A94

American Sociological Association, A95

American Thoracic Society, A96

American Veterinary Medical Association Film Library, A97

American Video Network, B10

Arco Publishing Co., Inc., G11

Arizona State University Media Research and Development, B11

Arkansas Department of Health, D3

Armed Forces Institute of Pathology, D4

Arnold Eagle Productions, B12

Aronson, see Jason Aronson, Inc., G40

Arthritis Foundation, A98

Aspect II Educational Films, B13

Association for Advancement of Behavior Therapy, A99

Association for the Advancement of Health Education, A100

Association of American Medical Colleges, A102

Association Films, see Schering Professional Film Library, F27

Association Instructional Materials, B14

Association of Mental Health Administrations, A103

Association of Military Surgeons of the U.S., A104

Association of Nervous and Former Mental Patients see Recovery, Inc.

Association of Operating Room Nurses, A105; see also American College of Surgeons Surgical Film Library

Association for the Study of Abortion, A101

Astra Pharmaceutical Products, Inc., F2

Athletic Institute, A106

Auburn University Library, E4

Audio Digest Foundation, B16

Audio Visual Associates, B17

Audiovisual Education in Neurosurgery see AVENS

Audio and Visual Methods Company, B15

Ayerst Laboratories, F3

BFA Educational Media, B30

Baker and Taylor Company, Audiovisual Services Division, B21

Ballen Booksellers International, C2

Ballinger Publishing Company, G12

Baltimore City Health Dept., D5

Bandera Enterprises, B22

Bartel Dental Book Company, Inc., G13

Basic Books, Inc., G14

Bausch & Lomb, Inc., F4

Baylor College of Medicine Film Library, B23

R.A., Becker, Inc., B24

Beckman New Dimensions, B25

Becton Dickinson & Co., Inc., F5; see also Clay Adams

Behavioral Research Laboratories, Inc., B26

Behavioral Sciences Tape Library, B27

Bellefaire Residential Treatment and Child Care Center, B28

Benchmark Films, B29

Berens International Eye Film Library, Inc., B59

Bicom Company, B31

Billy Budd Films, Inc., B32

Biomedical Engineering Society, A107

Bio Monitoring Applications, Inc., G15

P. & H. Bliss Company, C3

Blue Hill Educational System, Inc., B34

Bookpeople, C4

Boston University Medical Center, Office of Postgraduate Education, G16

R.R. Bowker Company, G17

Brady Company, B35

Brain Information Service, E5

Brigham Young University, Educational Media Services, B36

Brunner Mazel, G18

Bullfrog Films, B37

Bureau of Health Manpower, U.S. Public Health Service, D6

Burgess Publishing Company, G19

Burroughs Wellcome, Co., F6

Butler University Science Library, E6

Butterworths Professional and Educational Publishers, G20

CBS/Education and Publishing Group, B42

CFI—Counselor Films, Inc., B49

CRC Press, Inc., G23

CRM Productions, B64

California Medical Association see Audio-Digest

California Peace Officers' Association, A108

California State Department of Health, D27

Cambridge University Press, G21

Campbell Soup Co., F7

Campus Film Distributors, B38

Cancer Care, Inc., A109

Cancer Center, University of Texas see University of Texas Cancer Center

Career Aids, Inc., B39
Carmac Productions, B40
Carnation Research Laboratories, F8
Carolina Biological Supply Co., F9
Carousel Films, Inc., B41
Carr Foundation, A110
Case Western Reserve University Health Sciences Communication Center, B102
Catalog Publication Division, Library of Congress see Library of Congress Catalog Publication Division
Center of Alcohol Studies Rutgers University, H2
Center for Cassette Studies, B43
Center for Continuing Education in Podiatric Medicine, B44
Center for Disease Control, U.S. Public Health Service, Dept. of Health, Education and Welfare, D7
Center for Health Administration Studies, University of Chicago, H1
Center for Humanities, Inc., B45
Center for Mass Communications, B46
Centre Films, Inc., B47
Centron Educational Films, B48
Cereal Institute, Inc., A111
Chemical Abstracts Service, E7
Chemical Rubber Co., see CRC Press, G23
Chicago College of Osteopathic Medicine, Medical Library, E8
Child Welfare League of America, Inc., A112
Childbirth Without Pain Education Association, A113
Churchill Films, B50
Ciba Medical Education Division, F10
Cinema Concepts, B51
Clay Adams, B52
Cleveland Clinic Foundation, see Dept. of Artificial Organs, E13
The Cleveland Health Museum, B53
Cold Spring Harbor Laboratory, H3
College of American Pathologists, A114
College of Saint Teresa, Audio Visual Center, B54
Colorado State University Libraries, E9
Columbia Broadcasting System, see CBS, B42
Columbia University Press, see Center for Mass Communications, B46
Commonwealth Fund, A115
Communication Skills Corp., B55
Communications in Learning, B56
Concept Media, B57
Concordia Audiovisual Media, B58
Continuing Education in Neurological Sciences, B60

Convention of American Instructors of the Deaf, Inc., A116
Cook-Waite Laboratories, F11
Cornell University Educational Television Center, B61
Cornell University Medical College Library, E10
Cornell University Press, G22
Coronet Instructional Materials, B62
Council for Exceptional Children, A117
Council of Planning Librarians Exchange Bibliographies, A118
Counselor Films, Inc. see CF1
Countway Library of Medicine see Harvard University
Creative Learning Center, B63
Creighton University, Health Sciences Library, E11
Thomas Y. Crowell Co., Inc. see John Day, Abelard-Schuman
Curriculum Materials Corp., B65

Dana Biomedical Library see Dartmouth College
Dana Medical Library see University of Vermont
Dartmouth College, Dana Biomedical Library, E12
Datafilms, B66; see also Parthenon Pictures
Davidson Films, Inc., B67
F.A. Davis Company, G24
John Day, Abelard-Schuman, G25
Dayton Lab, B68
Defense Civil Preparedness Agency, The Pentagon, D8
Denar Corporation, F12
Denedco of Dallas, G26
Denoyer—Geppert Audiovisuals, B69
Department of Artificial Organs, Cleveland Clinic, E13
Devereux Foundation, A119
A.B. Dick Audio Visual Operations, B70
Direction South Media, B71
Division for the Blind and Physically Handicapped, Library of Congress see Library of Congress Div. for the Blind and Handicapped
Documatic Films, B72
Dover Publications, G27
Drug Abuse Council, A120
Drug, Chemical and Allied Trades Association, A121
Drug Intelligence Publications, G28
Drustar, Inc., B73
Dukane Corp., B74

Duke University Medical Center, Div. of Audiovisual Education, B75
Dunlap and Associates, Inc., F13

Eaton Medical Film Library, F14
Ebsco Subscription Services, C5
Spencer S. Eccles Medical Sciences Library *see* University of Utah
Edcoa Productions, B76
Educational Foundation of the American Society of Plastic and Reconstructive Surgeons, A122
Educational Innovators Press, B77
Educational Perspectives Associates, B78
Educational Products, Inc., B79
Educational Projections Corp., B80
Educational Resources Foundation, B81
Educational TV, B82
Educators Progress Service, G29
Eli Lilly and Company *see* Lilly
Eliot Books, C6
Elsevier/Excerpta Medica/North Holland, G30
Emcom, Inc., B83
Emphysema Anonymous, A123
Employers Insurance of Wausau, F15
Encyclopedia Britannica Educational Corp., B84
Environment Information Center, E14
Environmental Protection Agency *see* Air Pollution Technical Information Center
Epilepsy Foundation of America, A124
Euthanasia Educational Council, A125
Excerpta Medica Foundation, G31
Eye Gate House, B85

Fairchild Camera and Instrument Corp., B86
Falk Library of the Health Professions *see* University of Pittsburgh
Family Service Association of America, A126
Farm Film Foundation, B87
Federal Aviation Administration, D9
Fels Research Institute for the Study of Human Development, H4
Filmakers Library, Inc., B88
FIND—SVP Healthcare Information Center, E15
Florida State University, B89
Food and Drug Administration, D10
Foundation for Living, B90
Fox Chase Cancer Center, H5
Franciscan Films, B91

Futura Publishing Co., G32
Fye, W. Bruce, C7

GASP (Group Against Smog and Pollution), A127
Gale Research Co., G33
Geigy Pharmaceuticals, F16
General Services Administration *see* National Audiovisual Center
Georgia Regional Medical Television Network, B92
Gerontological Society, A128
Gilles de la Tourette Syndrome Association, A129
Glenn Educational Medical Services, Inc., B93
Gottesman Library *see* Albert Einstein College of Medicine
Graduate Program in Hospital and Health Administration, University of Iowa, H6
Graphic Films Corp., B94
Great Plains National Instructional Television Library, B95
Group for the Advancement of Psychiatry, A130
Group Against Smog and Pollution *see* GASP
Grune & Stratton, Inc. *see* Academic Press/
Guidance Associates/Harcourt, Brace Jovanovich, B96

Hallmark Films, B97
Harcourt Brace Jovanovich *see* Guidance Associates
Harper and Row Publishers, G34
Harris-Tuchman Productions, B98
Harvard University Francis A. Countway Library of Medicine, E16
Harvard University Press, G35
Hawaii State Department of Health, D11
Hay Fever Prevention Society, A131
Hazeldeu Rehabilitation Center *see* Emcom
Health Affairs Press, G36
Health Education Aids, B99
Health Education Programs, Inc., B100
Health Insurance Institute, E17
Health Management Systems, Inc., B101
Hiltz and Hayes Publishing Company, Inc., G37
Hoffman LaRoche *see* Roche Film Library; Rocom
Hogg Foundation for Mental Health, A133

Holden-Day, Inc., G38
Hospital Research and Educational Trust, B103
Howard University Medical Dental Library, E18
Human Factors Society, A135
Human Sciences Press, G39
Huxley Institute for Biosocial Research, A136

Idaho State University Library, E19
Illinois State Medical Society, A137
Illinois State University, Milner Library, E20
Industrial Health Foundation, A138
Information Center for Hearing, Speech and Disorders of Human Communications, E21
Insight Films—Paulist Productions, B104
Institute of Medicine, National Academy of Sciences, H7
Institute for the Study of Drug Misuse, A139
Instructional Dynamics, Inc., B105
International College of Applied Nutrition, A140
International Film Bureau, Inc., B106
International Library, Archives and Museum of Optometry, E22
International Nonwovens and Disposables Association, A141

Jason Aronson, Inc., G40
Jennie May Fels Memorial Library see Fels Research Institute for the Study of Human Development
Jeri Productions, B107
Johns Hopkins Medical Institutions see Information Center for Hearing, Speech, and Disorders of Human Communication
Johns Hopkins University, School of Hygiene and Public Health see American Journal of Epidemiology
Johns Hopkins University Welch Medical Library, E23
Johns Hopkins University Press, G41
Johns Hopkins University Press Audiovisual Division, B108
Johnson and Johnson, F17
Johnson Associates, Inc., G42
Johnson, Walter J., Inc., C8

Kansas Center for Mental Retardation and Human Development see Parsons State Hospital

Kansas State University Veterinary Medical Library, E24

La Leche League International, A142
Lalor Foundation, A143
Lane Medical Library see Stanford University School of Medicine
Lange Medical Publications, G43
Langley Porter Institute Library see University of California San Francisco
LaRue Films, Inc., see Scientificom, B152
Lawren Productions, Inc., B109
Lea & Febiger, G44
Learning Corporation of America, B110
Learning Dynamics, G45
Lexington Books, G46
Library of Congress Catalog Publication Division, D12
Library of Congress Division for the Blind, D13
Lilly Company, F18
Listening Library, Inc., B111
Lyman M. Stowe Library see University of Connecticut Health Center

MIT Press, G50
McGraw-Hill Films, B113
MacMillan Films, B112
Maine State Dept. of Health and Welfare see State of Maine Dept. of Health and Welfare
Massachusetts Institute of Technology see MIT Press, G50
Maternity Center Association, A144
Medical College of Wisconsin, Medical-Dental Library, E25
Medical Economics Company, G47
Medical Examination Publishing Co., Inc., G48
Medical Library Association, A145
Medical Library Center of New York, E26
Medical University of South Carolina, Dept. of Audiovisual Resources, B115
Medical University of South Carolina, Div. of Continuing Education, B116
Mended Hearts, A146
Mental Health Training Film Program, B117
Michigan Cancer Foundation, A147
Microcard Editions, G49
Milner-Fenwick, Inc., B118
Milton Roy Company, Ophthalmic Group, F19
Modern Talking Picture Service, B119
Mosby Company, G51
Mountain Plains Educational Media Council, B120

NTIS, *see* National Technical Information Service, E28

Narcotic Educational Foundation of America, A148

National Academy of Sciences, *see* Institute of Medicine, H7

National Agricultural Library, U.S. Dept. of Agriculture, D14

National Association for Hearing and Speech Action, A149

National Association for Mental Health, A150

National Association for Music Therapy, A151

National Association for Practical Nurse Education and Service, A152

National Association for Retarded Citizens, A153

National Association of Blue Shield Plans, A154

National Association of Chain Drug Stores, A155

National Association of Hospital Purchasing Management, A156

National Association of Residents and Interns, A157

National Audiovisual Center, D15

National Braille Association, A158

National Cancer Cytology Center, H8

National Cancer Foundation *see* Cancer Care

National Center for Audio Tapes, B121

National Center for Health Statistics, U.S. Public Health Service, D16

National Council on Aging, A159

National Easter Seal Society for Crippled Children and Adults, A160

National Environmental Health Association, A161

National Federation of Licensed Practical Nurses, A162

National Film Board of Canada, B122

National Foundation for Ileitis and Colitis, A163

National Foundation for Jewish Genetic Disease, A164

National Foundation for Sudden Infant Death, A165

National Foundation—March of Dimes, A166

National Genetics Foundation, A167

National Hemophilia Foundation, A168

National Information Center for Educational Media, E27

National Institute of Child Health and Human Development, D17

National Institute of Dental Research, D18

National Institutes of Health, D19; *see also* National Institute of Child Health and Human Development; National Institute of Dental Research

National Learning Corp., G52

National Library of Medicine, D20; *see also* National Medical Audiovisual Center

National Lupus Erythematosus Foundation, A169

National Medical Audiovisual Center, D21; *see also* National Library of Medicine

National Multiple Sclerosis Society, A170

National Public Relations Council of Health and Welfare Services, A171

National Rehabilitation Association, A172

National Safety Council, A173

National Society for the Prevention of Blindness, A174

National Technical Information Service, E28

National Women's Christian Temperance Union *see* Signal Press

New York Academy of Medicine Library, E29

New York State Health Department, D22

New York University Film Library, B123

North Carolina Safety Conference, A175

North Holland Publishing Company *see* Elsevier

Northwestern University Dental School Library, E30

Northwestern University *see* Prosthetic–Orthotic Center

Noyes Data Corporation, G53

Nutrition Foundation, A176

Nutrition Series, B124

Offenbacher, Old and Rare Books C9

Ohio River Valley Water Sanitation Commission, D23

Ohio State University, Dept. of Photography and Cinema, B125

Ohio State University Health Science Library, E31

Ohio State University Pharmacy Library, E32

Old Hickory Bookshop, C10

Ophthalmic Group, see Milton Roy Company, F19

Optical Society of America, A177

Orthopedic Audio Synopsis Foundation, B126

Orthopaedic Foundation *see* American Academy of Orthopaedic Surgeons

Orton Society, A178

O'Shea Books, C11

Oxford Films, B127

Parenteral Drug Association, A179

Parents' Magazine Films, Inc., B128

Parkinson's Disease Foundation, A180
Parsons State Hospital Media Support Services, B129
Parthenon Pictures/Datafilms, B130; *see also* Datafilms
Pennsylvania State University *see* Psychological Cinema Register
The Pentagon *see* Defense Civil Preparedness Agency
Perennial Education, Inc., B131
Personal Products Company, F20
Pfizer *see* Roering Division Film Library
Pharmaceuticals Manufacturers Association, A181
Phiebig, Inc., C12
Physicians Forum, A182
Physiological Training Company, B132
Pierre Fauchard Academy, A183
Planned Parenthood Foundation of America, A184
Polymorph Films, B133
Population Association of America, A185
Population Council, H9
Population Reference Bureau, A186
Prentice Hall, G54
President's Committee on Employment of the Handicapped, D24
Primary Medical Communications, B134
Princeton Microfilm Corp., G55
Princeton University Press, G56
Professional Arts, Inc., B135
Professional Information Library, B136
Professional Rehabilitation Workers With The Adult Deaf, A188
Professional Research, Inc., B137
Prosthetic–Orthotic Center, Northwestern University, H10
Psychodynamic Research Corp., B138
Psychological Cinema Register, B139
Psychological Films, Inc., B140
Public Affairs Committee, A188
Public Television Library, B141
Pyramid Films, B142

Q-Ed Productions, B143
Quintessence Publishing Co., Inc., G57

RMI Educational Films, Inc. Westwood Educational Productions, B146
Recovery, Inc., A189
Rehabilitation Institute of Chicago, H11
Rehabilitation International, A190
Rehabilitation Services Administration, D25
Rescue Breathing Film Associates, B144

Research Media, Inc., B145
Research Press, G58
Rittenhouse Book Distributors, Inc., C13
Robins Company, F21
Roche Film Library, F22
Rocom, F23
Roerig Division Film Library, F24
Ross Audio-Visual Library, F25
Ross Laboratories *see* Ross Audio-Visual Library
Routledge and Kegan Paul, G59
Roy Company *see* Milton Roy Company
Rush Medical College Library, E33
Rutgers University *see* Center of Alcohol Studies

SUNY Biomedical Communications Network *see* State University of New York
SUNY Stonybrook Health Sciences Library *see* State University of New York at Stonybrook
St. Louis Association for Retarded Children, A191
St. Luke's Hospital, B147
St. Martin's Press, G60
St. Paul Public Library, E34
Sandoz Pharmaceuticals, F26
Saturn Scientific, Inc., B148
Schaffer Library of the Health Sciences *see* Albany Medical College–Union Univ.
Schenkman Publishing Company, Inc., G61
Schering Professional Film Library, F27
Schloat Productions, B149
Schuman, Henry, Ltd., C14
W. Schwann, Inc., B150
Science and Health Publications, G62
Scientificom-Larue Communications, B151
G.D. Searle and Company, F28
Shell Film Library, F29
Signal Press, G63
Simon and Schuster, G64
Sister Kenny Institute, B152
Slack, Charles B., Inc., G65
Smart Family Foundation, A192
Smith, Kline and French Laboratories, F30
Smith, Miller and Patch, Inc., B153
Social and Rehabilitation Service, DHEW *see* Rehabilitation Services Administration
Social and Economic Statistics Administration, D26
Society of General Physiologists, A195
Society of Neurological Surgeons *see* AV-ENS
Society for Nutrition Education, A193
Society for Research in Child Development, A194

Society of Toxicology, A196
Society for Visual Education, Inc., B154
Soundwords, Inc., B155
Southern Illinois University, B156
Southern Medical Association, A197
Southern Regional Education Board, A198
Special Child Publications, G66
Special Libraries Association, A199
Spectrum Publications, Inc., G67
Spenco Medical Corporation, B157
Springer Publishing Co., G68
Springer-Verlag, G69
Squibb Medical Films, F31
Stanford University Medical Center, Lane
    Medical Library, E35
Stanton Films, B158
State Dept. of Health, California see Cali-
    fornia State Dept. of Health
State Dept. of Health, Hawaii see Hawaii
    State Dept. of Health
State Dept. of Health, New York see New
    York State Health Dept.
State of Maine Department of Health and
    Welfare, D28
State University of New York (SUNY)
    Biomedical Communications Network,
    E36
State University of New York at Stony-
    brook, Health Sciences Library, E37
Sterling Educational Films, B159
Stratton Intercontinental Medical Book
    Corp., G70
Stuart Finley, Inc., B160
Stuart Reynold Productions, B161
Sunburst Communications, B162
Sunkist Growers, Inc., F32
Syntex Laboratories, Inc., F33

TOPS Club (Take Off Pounds Sensibly),
    A200
Take Off Pounds Sensibly see TOPS Club,
    A200
Taplinger Publishing Co., Inc., G71
Teach 'Em, Inc., B163
Teachers College Press, G72
Teaching Films, Inc., B164
Telephone Lecture Network, B165
Telstar Productions, B166
Temple University Health Sciences Center,
    Dept. of Medical Communications,
    B167
C.S. Tepfer Publishing Company, Inc.,
    G73
Texas Women's University-College of Nurs-
    ing, B168
Three-M Company, B169
Time-Life Films, B170
Transaction Inc., G74

Tufts University Medical School-
    Educational Media Center, B171

Underwriters' Laboratories, H12
Union University see Albany Medical
    College-Union University, Schaffer
    Library
Unipub, G75
U.S. Army see Aeromedical Research Lab-
    oratory Library
U.S. Army see Armed Forces Institute of
    Pathology
U.S. Bureau of the Census, Dept. of Com-
    merce see Social and Economic Statis-
    tics Administration
U.S. Department of Agriculture see Na-
    tional Agriculture Library
U.S. Dept. of Commerce see National Tech-
    nical Info. Service; Social and Eco-
    nomic Statistics Administration
U.S. Food and Drug Administration see
    Food and Drug Administration
U.S. Dept. of Health, Education and Wel-
    fare, U.S. Public Health Service, see
    Bureau of Health Manpower; Center
    for Disease Control; National Center
    for Health Statistics; National Institute
    of Child Health and Human Develop-
    ment; National Institute of Dental
    Research; National Institutes of
    Health; National Library of Medicine;
    National Medical Audiovisual Center;
    Rehabilitation Services Administration
U.S. Dept. of Transportation see Federal
    Aviation Administration
U.S. Public Health Service, Dept. of
    Health, Education and Welfare see
    Bureau of Health Manpower; Center
    for Disease Control; National Center
    for Health Statistics; National Library
    of Medicine; National Medical Audio-
    visual Center
Universal Education and Visual Arts, B172
University of Alabama School of Dentistry,
    B173
University of Arizona—Arizona Medical
    Center, B174
University of California Berkeley Education
    Psychology Library, E38
University of California Extension Media
    Center, B175
University of California at Los Angeles
    Biomedical Library see Brain Informa-
    tion Service
University of California at Los Angeles,
    Medical Media Network, B114
University of California Press, G76
University of California, San Francisco

Educational TV Division *see* Educational TV

University of California San Francisco, Langley Porter Neuropsychiatric Library, E39

University of California, San Francisco Library, E40

University of Chicago *see* Center for Health Administration Studies

University of Chicago Press, G77

University of Connecticut, Center for Instructional Media and Technology, B176

University of Connecticut Health Center, Biomedical Communications, B177

University of Connecticut Health Center, Lyman Maynard Stowe Library, E41

University of Hawaii School of Public Health Library, E42

University of Illinois Press, G78

University of Iowa, B178

University of Iowa *see* Graduate Program in Hospital and Health Administration

University of Iowa Health Science Library, E43

University of Maine Film Rental Library, B179

University of Michigan Audio-Visual Education Center, B180

University of Michigan Chemistry-Pharmacy Library, E44

University of Michigan Public Health Library, E45

University of Minnesota Press, G79

University of Missouri, Columbia Medical Library, E46

University of Missouri Press, G80

University of Nebraska Medical Center, Library of Medicine, E47

University of Nebraska, Omaha, Biomedical Communications Center, B33

University of New Hampshire, New England Health Resources Center, B181

University of New Mexico Health Sciences Library, E48

University of North Carolina School of Medicine, Medical Television Center, B182

University of North Carolina School of Medicine Self-Instructional Materials Project, B183

University of Oregon Health Sciences Library, E49

University of Pennsylvania Press, G81

University of Pittsburgh Falk Library of the Health Professions, E50

University Presses of Florida, G83

University of South Dakota School of Medicine Health Science Library, E51

University of Southern California *see* National Information Center for Educational Media

University of Texas Cancer Center, M.D. Anderson Hospital Research Medical Library, E52

University of Texas Health Science Center at San Antonio, B184

University of Utah, Spencer S. Eccles Medical Sciences Library, E53

University of Vermont, Charles A. Dana Medical Library, E54

University of Wisconsin Press, G82

University of Wyoming Audio Visual Services *see* Mountain Plains Educational Media Council

University of Wyoming Film Library, B185; *see also* Mountain Plains Educational Media Council

Upjohn Company, F34

Vanderbilt University Medical Center Library, E55

Vanderbilt University Press, G84

Viking Press, G85

Ward's Natural Science Establishment, F35

Washington University School of Medicine Library, E56

Wayne State University, B186

Wayne State University Press, G86

Welch Medical Library *see* Johns Hopkins University

Western Psychological Services, G87

Westwood Educational Productions *see* RMI

Wexler Film Productions, Inc., B187

Wiley Biomedical Division, G88

Williams and Wilkins Co., G89

H.W. Wilson Co., G90

World Health Organization *see* American Association for World Health, Inc.

Xerox Education Publications/Xerox Films, B188

Xerox University Microfilms, G91

Yale Medical Library, E57

Yankee Book Peddler, C15

Year Book Medical Publishers, Inc., G92

Zero Population Growth, A201

Index to Free or Inexpensive Material

Alexander Graham Bell Association, A5
Allergy Foundation of America, A6
American Academy of Pediatrics, A18
American Association of Colleges of Pharmacy, A26
American Association of Dental Schools, A27
American Association for Maternal and Child Health, A20
American Association of Orthodontists, A30
American Association of Sex Educators and Counselors, A31
American Cancer Society, A34
American College Health Association, A37
American College of Nurse-Midwives, A39
American College of Radiology, A40
American College of Surgeons, A41
American Corrective Therapy Association, A44
American Council on Alcohol Problems, A45
American Dental Association, A46
American Diabetes Association, A48
American Foundation for the Blind, A49
American Heart Association, A52
American Hospital Association, A53
American Institute of the History of Pharmacy, A55
American Lung Association, A57
American Medical Association, A58
American Medical Technologists, A61
American Medical Women's Association, A62
American Natural Hygiene Society, A63
American Optometric Association, A65

American Osteopathic Association, A67
American Physical Therapy Association, A69
American Podiatry Association, A71
American Protestant Hospital Association, A73
American Social Health Association, A79
American Society of Internal Medicine, A93
Arkansas Department of Health, D3
Arthritis Foundation, A98
Association for the Advancement of Health Education, A100
Association of Operating Room Nurses, A105
Association for the Study of Abortion, A101
Athletic Institute, A106

Baltimore City Health Dept., D5
Bureau of Health Manpower, U.S. Public Health Service, D6

California State Department of Health, D27
Cancer Care, Inc., A109
Center for Disease Control, U.S. Public Health Service, Dept. of Health, Education and Welfare, D7
Cereal Institute, Inc., A111
Child Welfare League of America, Inc., A112
Childbirth Without Pain Education Association, A113

Defense Civil Preparedness Agency, The
    Pentagon, D8
Drug Abuse Council, A120

Emphysema Anonymous, A123
Employers Insurance of Wausau, F15
Epilepsy Foundation of America, A124
Euthanasia Educational Council, A125

Family Service Association of America,
    A126
Federal Aviation Administration, D9
Food and Drug Administration, D10
Fox Chase Cancer Center, H5

Gilles de la Tourette Syndrome Association,
    A129

Hawaii State Department of Health, D11
Hay Fever Prevention Society, A131
Health Insurance Institute, E17
Huxley Institute for Biosocial Research,
    A136

International College of Applied Nutrition,
    A140

Johnson and Johnson, F17

La Leche League International, A142
Library of Congress Division for the Blind,
    D13

Maternity Center Association, A144
Mended Hearts, A146
Michigan Cancer Foundation, A147
Milton Roy Company, Ophthalmic Group,
    F19

Narcotic Educational Foundation of Amer-
    ica, A148
National Association for Hearing and
    Speech Action, A149
National Association for Mental Health,
    A150
National Association for Practical Nurse
    Education and Service, A152
National Association for Retarded Citizens,
    A153
National Association of Blue Shield Plans,
    A154

National Braille Association, A158
National Center for Health Statistics, U.S.
    Public Health Service, D16
National Easter Seal Society for Crippled
    Children and Adults, A160
National Federation of Licensed Practical
    Nurses, A162
National Foundation for Ileitis and Colitis,
    A163
National Foundation for Sudden Infant
    Death, A165
National Foundation—March of Dimes,
    A166
National Genetics Foundation, A167
National Hemophilia Foundation, A168
National Institute of Child Health and
    Human Development, D17
National Institute of Dental Research, D18
National Institute of Health, D19
National Lupus Erythematosus Founda-
    tion, A169
National Multiple Sclerosis Society, A170
National Public Relations Council of
    Health and Welfare Services, A171
National Safety Council, A173
National Society for the Prevention of
    Blindness, A174
New York State Health Department, D22
Nutrition Foundation, A176

Orton Society, A178

Parkinson's Disease Foundation, A180
Personal Products Company, F20
Pharmaceuticals Manufacturers Associa-
    tion, A181
Physicians Forum, A182
Planned Parenthood Foundation of Amer-
    ica, A184
Public Affairs Committee, A188

Recovery, Inc., A189
Ross Audio-Visual Library, F25

St. Louis Association for Retarded Chil-
    dren, A191
Shell Film Library, F29
State of Maine Department of Health and
    Welfare, D28

Underwriters' Laboratories, H12

Zero Population Growth, A201

Subject Index

Abortion, A101, A186, G37, G68
Accident prevention *see* Safety
Accidents, A18
Acupuncture, A38, B7, B44, B112, B142, G29
 see also Asian medicine; Chinese medicine
Addiction, drug *see* Drug abuse
Administration, A25, B116, D22, G12, H6
 family services, A126
 health, A12, B178, G46, H1
 hospital, A53, A73, A83, A156, B56, G62
 medical staff, B163
 mental health, A103
 pharmacy, A26
 see also Management
Adolescents, A80, B96, B109, B110, B112, B119, G18
Adoption, A112
Aerospace medicine *see* Medicine, aerospace
Aged, A118, A128, A190, D75, G68, G83
 see also Aging; Gerontology
Aging, A118, A130, A186, B106, A159, B46, B61, D17, F7
 see also Aged; Gerontology
Agriculture, D14
Air pollution *see* Pollution, air
Alcohol *see* Drug abuse; Alcoholism; Drinking
Alcoholism, A4, A33, A45, A58, A74, A136, A139, A154, B83, B85, B90, B138, B141, B156, G12, G59, H2
 treatment facilities, A4
 see also Drinking
Allergies, A6, A8, B5, F27
 see also Asthma, Hay fever

Allergy clinics
 list of, A6
Allied health, A88, B55, B145, D6, G32, G34, G68, G88
 see also specific field
Anatomy, B31, B35, B50, B52, B53, B65, B69, B80, B85, B99, B120, B125, B148, B157, B164, B166, B178, B180, F9, F10, G4, G11, G34, G44
Anemia
 sickle cell, B63
Anesthesia, F11
Animals, A97
Anthropology, B139, B138, F9
Aphasia, A5, A149, G4
Architectural barriers, A160, A190
Arthritis, A98
Artificial organs, E13
Asian medicine, E16
 see also Acupuncture; Chinese medicine
Asthma, A6, A57
 see also Allergies
Athletics *see* Physical fitness; Sports
Audiology, A5
Audiovisual materials
 information, B24
 management of, D21, E27, G17
 production of, B11
Autism, A117, B141, G58
Aviation medicine *see* Medicine, aerospace

Back issues of journals *see* Journal, back issues
Backache, A37
Bacteriology, A84
Behavior, B14, B26, B29, B123, G45, G58,

G66, G74
animal, B139
psychomotor, B77
Behavior modification, B64, B97, B145
Behavior therapy see Therapy, behavior
Bioanalysis, A24
Biochemistry, A35, B55, B149, G4, G5, G9,
    G39, G69, G83, H4
Biocommunication, A133
Biofeedback, G17
Biology, B1, B4, B26, B29, B41, B45, B52,
    B62, B64, B69, B70, B84, B111, B112,
    B120, B122, B127, B146, B148, B149,
    B170, B172, B179, B180, B185, B188,
    F9, G1, G2, G6, G9, G19, G21, G25,
    G27, G30, G34, G67, G69, G76, G78,
    G79, G81, G83
    molecular, H3
Biology specimens, F35
Birth control, B63, F9
    see also Family planning; Abortion
Birth defects, A166
Birth rates, A186
Blindness, A48, A158, A174, B5, D25, G66
    see also Handicapped
Blood see Hematology
Blood donation, A25
Blood Pressure, A52, G18
Blood transfusion, A25
Bloom's Syndrome, A164
Book reviews, C15
Books
    foreign, C1, C12
    out of print, C7, C11, C12
    rare, C7, C9, C10, C14, E12
    see also specific subject
Braille materials, A142, A158, D13, G9
Brain, E5
Breast feeding, A20, A142, B133, F25
Breast self-examination, A147
Breathing, A123

Camps, A191, B117
Cancer, A19, A34, A41, A109, A147, B57,
    D17, E52, F34, G68, H5, H8
Cardiology, A38, G70
Cardiovascular disease, A38
Cardiovascular system, A42
Cardiovascular disease, A52, B19, B151,
    B155, F1
Career information, B49, B113, B120
    allied health, A88
    bacteriology, F5
    chiropractory, A36
    dental hygiene, A47
    dentistry, A27

health sciences, A118, B30, B35, B48,
    B62, B188, G29, G71
hospital administration, A135
medical assistants, A61
medical technology, A61
medicine, A62, A102, B121
music therapy, A151
nursing, A39, A105, A162
orthodontics, A30
osteopathy, A67
pharmacy, A26
podiatry, A71
practical nursing, A152
rehabilitation, A160
Catalogs, D12
Cataracts, A174
Catheters, F6
Cerebrovascular disease, A52, B57, B152
    nursing care, B81
Chaplains, A53, A73, B56, G40
Chemical industry, A121
Chemicals, A86
Chemistry, A35, B69, B84, E7, G4, G34,
    G53
Child abuse, A112, A117, B5, B112, G59
Child care, A29, A58, A142, A144, A184,
    A188, B106, F17, F25, G39
    see also Pediatrics; Health, child
Child development, A157, A195, B61, B67,
    B97, B125, B128, B139, D17, G39, G77,
    H4
Childbirth, B10, B47, B70, B88, B109, B128,
    B131, B172, G60, G71
    natural, A113, A144, B63, B133
Child Development, B123
Children, A126, A130, B28, B38, B128,
    D17, G72
    emotionally disturbed, A119
    exceptional, A117
Chinese medicine, H7
    see also Asian medicine; Acupuncture
Chiropractory, A36
City of Hope, A169
Civil defense, D8
Cleft palate, D18
Colitis, A163
College health service, A37
Colostomy, A147, B152
Communicable disease see Infectious dis-
    ease
Communications, A171
Community mental health, A153, G39, G68,
    G86
Community services, A170
Computers, A54, A57
Consumer information, D10
Contact lenses, B66, F19
Continuing education, B171

allergy, A8
allied health, B165
dentistry, B165
medical records, A59
medical technologists, A61
medicine, A67, A89, B10, B16, B24, B82,
    B108, B116, B165
nursing, A105, A165, B152, B165
neurology, B60
nutrition, A140
ophthalmology, A13
orthopedics, A16
osteopathy, A17, A67
otolaryngology, A13
pathology, A89, A114
physiology, A70
podiatry, B44, B165
surgery, A87
veterinary, A97
Contraception see Family planning
Coronary care, B116
Cost analysis, H6
Cost of education, H7
Cost of health care, A182
Counseling, A167, A191, B38, B106, B129,
    G5, G87
cancer, A109
family planning, A184
genetic, A167
marriage, A31, B105
patient, B118, B137
sex, A31, B76, B82
Crib death see Sudden infant death
Crippled children and adults, A167
Crisis intervention, B35, B138

Dance, A100
Day care, A112, A119, A153, G39
Deafness, A5, A116, A117, A149, A188,
    A190, E21, G66
Death, A125, B5, B32, B78, B88, B112,
    B162, G39
Death rates, A186
Delinquency see Juvenile delinquency
Delivery of health care see Health care
    delivery
Demography, A186
Dental assisting, B118
Dental hygiene, A47, G4
Dental schools, A27
Dentistry, A10, A15, A27, A30, A46, A47,
    B56, B102, B173, B178, C6, D6, D15,
    D17, D21, F2, F11, F12, G13, G26,
    G44, G51, G57, G89, G92, H4
preventive, B19
Dermatology, F18, F27
Diabetes, A48, B118, B155, F7, F34, G71

in pregnancy, G84
Diagnosis, B109, B125, B187, F1, F18
Diet, A63, A136, A200, B10, B37, B62, B65,
    B122, G11, G17, G29, G71
diabetic, A48
see also Nutrition
Dietary department, A53, G19
Digestion, F7
Disasters, D8
Disease, B121, D3, F16
infectious, A18, A58, B5, D5, D7, G7
West African, D7
see also specific disease
Disease transmission, D7
Disposable equipment, A141
Divorce, A185
Doctors see Physicians
Down's Syndrome, B141, B174, D17
Drinking, A45, A58, A154, B2, B8, B36,
    B63, B96, B112, B113, B127, B131,
    B142, B157, B178, G63, H2
see also Alcoholism
Drug abuse, A4, A33, A45, A48, A100,
    A108, A120, A133, A136, A139, A148,
    A154, A181, A188, B1, B5, B6, B7, B8,
    B14, B29, B35, B41, B46, B50, B53,
    B58, B61, B83, B85, B104, B106, B111,
    B112, B121, B127, B129, B131, B135,
    B138, B141, B143, B154, B162, B170,
    B178, D5, G12, G61, G63, G74
Drug evaluation, A68
Drug information, A78, A92
Drug stores, A155
Drugs, A68, A179, D10, F1, F18, F21, F33,
    G53
cost of, A182
illicit, A33
manufacture, A121, A181
parenteral, A179
Dysantonomia, A164
Dyslexia, A178
Dystonia, A164

Ecology, B62, B84, B122, B142, B160, B172,
    E7
Education, B176
chemical, A35
childbirth, A113
deaf, A116
dental, A27, A183
environmental health, A161
health, A100
health professionals, B75, B79
health sciences, A133, A198, B15
hospital purchasing, A156
medical, A29, A60, A102, A115, A130,
    A182, H6

music therapy, A151
nurses' aides, B73
nursing, A28, A39, A105, B10, B54, B57
nutrition, A193
parent, A144, A160
patient, A192
pharmacy, A26
physical see Physical Fitness
plastic and reconstructive surgery, A122
practical nursing, A152
radiology, A40
sex, A31, A58, A78, A79, A100, A112,
    A133, A188, B53, B58, B82, B97, B131,
    B154, G17, G37
special, G78
see also Continuing Education; Sexuality
Elderly see Aged
Electrosurgery, A10
Embryology, B94
Emergency care, A16, A108, B35, B100,
    B118, B144, B163, D8
Emphysema, A123
Employment information see Placement in-
    formation
Endoscopy, A82
Engineering, A94
    biomedical, A107, D1, E13
Entomology, A94
Environment, B29, E14, G41, G53, G74
Environmental health see Health, Environ-
    mental
Epidemiology, G7
Epilepsy, A124
Ethics, A125
Euthanasia, A125, B112
Examination review books, G11, G48, G52
Exercise, B62, B85, B158, G86
Eye diseases, A174
Eye safety, F4
Eyes, A65, B10, B19, B29, B125, B137, D17,

Families, B61, B72, B96, B106, B128, B131,
    G5, G39, G59
Family planning, A31, A184, A185, B19,
    B8, B66, B122, B127, B130, B131,
    B157, H9
see also Contraception; Abortion
Family practice, B10
Family services, A109, A112, A126, A129,
    A166, A170, A191
Family therapy, G58
Fasting, A63
Feet, A71
Fertility, A184, G86
Films
    production, A16

Financial counseling, A72
Financial management, A135, G47
First aid, A188, B42, B8, B9, B35, B80, B85,
    B120, B142, B144, B156, B162, B179,
    G19, G29, G86
Fitness see Physical fitness
Flu, A57, D7
Food, D10, D14, E7, F8, G53
Food technology, B55
Foreign medical graduates, A29
Foreign language materials, A6, A41, A57,
    A146, A166, A184, A188, A190, B72,
    A79, B84, B89, B106, B127, B143,
    B161, C1, F20, G37, G43, H9
Forensic Sciences, A11, A86, B136
Fractures see Orthopedics
Fund raising, A171

Gastroenterology, A163, G70
Gaucher's Disease, A164
Genetic disease, A164, A166, A167
Genetics, A25, B45, B118, B120, G2, G34,
    G41, G44, H3
Gerontology, A128, G83
    see also Aged
Gilles de la Tourette Syndrome, A129
Glaucoma, A174
Group dynamics, B105
Group practice, A50
Group therapy, A189
Growth, B169, B178, D3, D17, F20, G72
Gynecology, B187

HMOs see Health maintenance organiza-
    tions
Halfway houses, A74
Handicapped, A6, A160, A172, B38, B131,
    B152, D13, D24
    see also specific handicap
Handicapped children, A117
Hay fever, A6, A131, B155, F1
    see also Allergies
Health, B1, B4, B26, B32, B35, B36, B45,
    B70, B74, B85, B95, B111, B127, B154,
    B159, B178, B185, B186, C4, D3, D15,
    D17, D22, F15, F18, G3, G9, G11,
    G29, G34, G36, G73
    child, A78, F25
    dental, A30, A46, A47
    environmental, A127, A41, A77, A161,
        B46
    industrial, A138
    maternal, A20, A58, A118, A144, F7,
        F25, B156
    mental, A32, A78, A103, A133, A150,
        A189, B3, B35, B36, B41, B106, B117,

B122, B131, B154, G12, G29
personal, A58, A77
school, A18, A39, A78
social, A79
world, A23
see also Child care; Pediatrics
Health care delivery, A50, A103, A118,
   A182, B14, B141, G35, G39
   religious, A73
Health care policy, G82
Health education see Education, health
Health maintenance organizations, A50, H7
Health manpower, A198, D6, D25
Hearing aids, A149
Hearing disorders see Deafness
Heart, B42, B46, B142, D17
Heart disease see Cardiovascular disease
Heart sounds, B132
Heart surgery, A146
Hematology, A25, A90, F26, G34
Hemophilia, A90, A168
Hepatitis, A25, D7, F1
History
   of dentistry, E30
   of health sciences, D19
   of health sciences, E50
   of medicine, B106, B136, C7, C14, D20,
      D21, E10, E29, E35, G10, G22, G27,
      G41, G56, G71, G76, G82
   of nursing, B166
   of pharmacy, A55, E44
   of psychiatry, B117
   of psychology, G14
   see also Books, rare
Homosexuality, A188, B131
Hospital administration see Administra-
   tion, hospital
Hospital trustees, B103
Hospitalization, involuntary, A21
Hospitals, A53, A73, A91, A83, A92, A135,
   A141, B13, B181, F2
   cost of, A182
Human factors, A135
Hygiene, A94, B26, B36, B62, B65, B69,
   B80, B84, B89, B111, B119, B120,
   B121, B127, B137, B154, B158, B169,
   B178, B180, B185, D5, D22, F17, G9,
   G29
   dental, A47
   natural, A63
   personal, B6
Hyperactivity, A136, G29
Hypertension see Blood pressure

Ileitis, A163
Ileostomy, B152
Immunology, A9, A25, A84, G35, G38
Indexes, D20, G90

Industrial safety see Safety
Influenza see Flu
Information searches, E15
Inhalation therapy, A53
Inherited disease see Genetic disease
Injection techniques, F5
Instrumentation, A54, G2
Insurance, E17, H6,
   group, A93
   health, A154, G2
   national health, A182
Internal medicine see Medicine, internal
International health see World health
Interns, A157
Intestinal diseases see Gastroenterology

Jews, A31
   genetic disease, A164
Job information see Placement information
Journals
   back issues, C3, C8
   foreign, C5, C12
   subscriptions, C3, C5, C6, C12
Juvenile delinquency, A133, G87

L-dopa, A180
L.S.D. see Drug abuse
Laboratories, A24, A25, A61, A84, A86,
   A89, A114, B187, G44
Laboratory equipment, F5
Laboratory technique, B25, B55, G34
Lamaze-Pavlov childbirth, A113, B133
   see also Childbirth, natural
Language, E21
Law, A11, A21, A33, A83, A91, A101,
   A117, A125, A130, B136, F22, G62
   dental hygiene, A47
   medical practice, A50
   nursing, A39
   see also Medicine, forensic; Malpractice
Law enforcement, A108
Learning, B38, B40, B110, D17, G34, G66,
   G72
Learning disabilities, A117, A136, A160,
   A178, B109
Legal assistance, A21
Librarianship, A56, B56
Libraries, A118, A199
   medical, A145
Licensed practical nurses, A152
Legislation see Law
Licensed Practical Nurses, A162
Life Science see Biology
Lipreading, A6, A149
Longevity, E12
Lung disease see Respiratory disease

Lungs, D17
Lupus erythematosus, A169

Malaria, D7
Malpractice, A50, G47
    see also Law
Mammography, A40
Management, A12, A72, B101, B163, G47
    financial, A135, A157
    of health care, G67
    personnel, A83
    see also Administration, Practice Man-
    agement
Manpower see Health manpower
Marijuana see Drug abuse
Marriage, A184, A185, B58, B97, B128,
    B162, G37, G39, G58, G74, G87
Materials testing, A86
Maternal health see Health, maternal
Measles, D7
Media see Audiovisual materials
Medical assistants, A61
Medical education see Education, medical
Medical records, A59
Medical research, D19
Medical school see Education, medical;
    Students, medical
Medical sociology, G67
Medical technology, A61, A89
Medical terminology see Terminology,
    medical
Medication, F11
Medicine, A197, B22, B23, B33, B42, B56,
    B71, B82, B86, B89, B92, B93, B98,
    B102, B109, B114, B134, B136, B139,
    B147, B153, B167, B168, B171, B175,
    B177, B178, B182, B183, B184, B186,
    C1, C2, C6, C13, D6, D15, F2, F3, F6,
    F14, F20, F26, F28, F31, G1, G12,
    G21, G24, G25, G30, G32, G35, G41,
    G43, G47, G51, G67, G68, G69, G70,
    G76, G77, G78, G79, G80, G81, G88,
    G89, G92
    aerospace, A3, A114, D1
    forensic, A33, B136
    industrial, A138
    internal, A7, A82, A93, B10, F1, F18,
    G34
    laboratory, A84, A85
    military, A104
    nuclear, B25, G75
    preventive, B19
    psychosomatic, A1
    rehabilitation, A43
    tropical, A94
    see also Veterinary medicine
Meningitis, D7

Menstruation, B122, F20
Mental health see Health, mental; Mental
    illness
Mental illness, A108, A150, A159, B7, B8,
    B28, B109, B112, B138, F1, G59
    rehabilitation, A119
    see also Schizophrenia; Health, mental
Mental retardation, A18, A117, A119,
    A153, A188, A191, B14, B97, B129,
    B133, B160, D25, G39, G58, G89
    see also specific condition
Methadone, B5
Microbiology, B120, B166, B178, B179,
    D15, G19
Microform publications, G49, G55, G75,
    G91
Microscopy, B41, F4, F34
Midwifery, A39, A144
Military medicine, A104
Mongolism see Down's Syndrome
Multiple sclerosis, A170
Mumps, D7
Music therapy, A151

National health service, A182
Natural childbirth see Childbirth, natural
Natural foods, A63
Neoplasms see Cancer
Neurobiology, G2
Neurology, A180, B60, B82, B136, E5, F27,
    G68, G70
Neuropsychiatry, E40
Neurosurgery, B20
Niemann-Pick Disease, A164
Noise, B6
Nurse-midwives, A39
Nurses, A39
    doctors' office, A28
    practical, A152, A162
    private duty, A162
    vocational, A152, A162
Nurses' aides, B73
Nursing, A198, B12, B34, B35, B36, B39,
    B41, B54, B56, B57, B81, B98, B99,
    B106, B114, B120, B145, B166, B168,
    B178, B186, C6, D6, D21, F30, G8,
    G11, G19, G24, G34, G47, G51, G54,
    G65, G68, G72, G73, G82, G88, G89
    hospital, A53
    operating room, A42, A105
    psychiatric, B161
    tropical medicine, A94
Nutrition, A18, A20, A58, A63, A110,
    A111, A142, A166, A176, A186, A193,
    B6, B21, B29, B35, B37, B51, B61, B84,
    B85, B87, B89, B96, B113, B119, B124,
    B125, B143, B154, B156, B158, B162,

B169, B178, B179, D14, D18, F7, F18, F25, F32, G11, G16, G29, G60, G64, G75, G84
applied, A140
world, F29, G75
see also Diet

Obesity, B14, B41, B155, B156, B157, G60
Obstetrics, A39, B82, F26
Occlusion, F12
Operating room technique, A42
Opthalmology, A13, B59
Optics, A177
Optometry, A14, A65, A198, E22
Oral hygiene, A30, A46, B36, B53, B65, B113, B118, B122, B124, B137, D159, B178, D18
Orthodontics, A30
Orthomolecular therapy see Vitamin therapy
Orthopedics, A16, B21, B44, B126, B187
Orthopsychiatry, A66
Osteopathy, A17, A67, E8, H4
Otolaryngology
videotapes, A13

Pacemakers, B98
Parenteral drugs, A179
Prenatal care, A166
Pariasitology, A94, G34
Parkinson's Disease, A180
Pastoral care see Chaplains
Pathology, A89, A114, B94, B148, B175, B178, D4, D21, F10
oral, A15
Patient care, B10, F18, F33
Pediatrics, A18, B82, F25, F26, G84
see also Children
Personal development, B105, B111
Pesticides, F29
Pharmaceuticals see Drugs
Pharmacology, A81, A85, B136, B166, B187, G4
applied, A196
Pharmacy, A26, A68, A92, A155, B116, B130, C6, E44, G19, G28, G89
Physical education see Physical fitness
Physical examination, B71
Physical fitness, A58, A63, A100, A106, A119, B80, B84, B107, B111, B172, G6, G11, G19, G29, G64
Physical therapy see Therapy, physical
Physicians
foreign medical graduates, A29
women, A62
Physics, A54

Physiology, A70, A195, B85, B99, B149, F10, G2, G11, G21, G34
Placement information
alcoholism treatment, A4
hospital purchasing, A156
music therapy, A154
overseas, A23
physicians, A50
psychology, A76
Planning, A118, H6
health services, F13
regional, A198
Podiatry, A71
Poisoning, A18, B2, B5, B63
food, D10
see also Toxicology
Police, A108
Policy
health care, G82
Pollution, B1, B110, B160, D23
air, A57, A127, B41, E1, F29
environmental, A127
Population, A110, A185, A186, A188, A201, B45, B66, G12, H9
Practical management, A40, A50, A72, A93, F16, F23, G47
Pregnancy, A20, A142, A144, A167, B19, B48, B72, B109, B128, B141
Prosthetics, H10
Psychopharmacology, G67
Psychosomatic medicine see Medicine, psychosomatic
Psychotherapy, A130, B82, G39, G64
group, A51
Public affairs, G12, G14
Public health, A77, A118, A190, B168, D2, D3, D22, G22, G35, G41, G68, G73, G74, G82, H1
Public relations, A40, A53
Publications, A171
Purchasing
hospital, A156

Rabies, D7
Radiology, A40, B82, D15, G4, G16, G75
standards, A86
Rat control, D5
Records, medical see Medical records
Recreation, A106
for handicapped, A160
for mentally retarded, A153, A191
Rehabilitation, A43, A160, A172, A188, A190, B83, B90, B125, B129, B152, B175, B178, D21, D25, G78, H10, H11
Reprints, C8, C11, G27, G77, H4
Reproduction, B70, B122, B148, B149
Residents, A157

Respiratory disease, A57, A96, B155, G60
  see also specific disease
Respiratory therapy, B93
Resuscitation, B144
Retardation see Mental retardation
Rheumatic fever, F1
Rheumatism, A98
Right-to-die, A125
Ringworm, D7

S.L.E., A169
Safety, A20, A100, A108, A160, A173,
  A175, A188, B1, B2, B4, B9, B50, B66,
  B74, B80, B84, B111, B122, B135,
  B142, B185, D1, D3, D9, D15, F4,
  G29, G73, H12
  eye, A174
  occupational, B130, F15
Sanitation, D8
School health see Health, school
Schizophrenia, A136, F25, G14
Science, A22, B69, B121, G25, G29, G30,
  G50
Scientific handbooks, G23
Self-assessment examinations see Examina-
  tion review books
Self-examination
  breast, A147
Self-help, A189
Sex education see Education, sex
Sex roles, B29
Sexuality, A31, A184, A191, B27, B32, B61,
  B70, B76, B85, B104, B111, B118,
  B140, B141, B142, B143, B146, B155,
  B159, F20, G34, G39, G58, G64, G70,
  G87
  see also Education, sex
Sickle cell anemia, B63
Sleep, E5
Smog see Pollution, air
Smoking, A2, A28, A45, A57, A58, A139,
  A147, B6, B10, B14, B36, B48, B53,
  B96, B109, B112, B113, B122, B141,
  B142, B157, G63
Social welfare, A171
Social work, A126
Sociology, A95
Space medicine see Medicine, aerospace
Spanish language materials see Foreign
  language materials
Spectometry, A86
Speech, A178, E21, G34, G78, G87
Speech pathology, B27
Speech therapy, A6, A149, B107
Sports, A106
  injuries, B9, B112
  see also Physical fitness

Standards, A86
  professional, A102
Statistics, D6, D7, D16, D26, E17, G7, H1
  population, A186
Sterile products, A179
Sterilization
  reproductive, A184
Stroke see Cerebrovascular disease
Students, A157
  medical, A60
Stuttering, A149
Subscriptions see Journals, subscriptions
Sudden infant death, A165, D17
Suicide, A32, A154, A188, B35, B138, G39
  prevention centers, A32
Surgery, A41, A42, A105, B10, B23, B44,
  B71, B82, B125, B126, B151, B178,
  B187, F1, F18, F27, F34, G35
  abdominal, A87
  films, A7
  heart, A146
  nervous system, B20
  orthopedic, A16
  plastic and reconstructive, A122
Surgical supplies, A141

Tay-Sachs Disease, A164
Technologists
  medical, A61
  X-ray, A40
Teeth, D123
  see also Oral hygiene
Television, instructional, B3
Terminology, medical, B18, B21
Tests, A86
  psychological, A66
Tetanus, D7
Therapy
  behavior, A74, A99
  family, G58
  gestalt, B43
  group, A189, G18
  music, A151
  occupational, B56
  physical, A69, B56, G19
  respiratory, B93
  sex, A31
  see also Psychotherapy
Thoracic disease, A96
Tooth care see Oral hygiene
Tourette Syndrome, A129
Toxicology, A138, A196, B174
  see also Poisoning
Trauma, B151
Trustees, B103
Transactional analysis, B105

Transplantation, F34
Tuberculosis, A57, B63

Urban health, G68
Urinalysis, G34

V.D. *see* Venereal disease
Vasectomy, B141
Venereal disease, A45, A58, A63, A79, B1,
    B6, B8, B19, B26, B35, B46, B48, B50,
    B53, B63, B69, B85, B91, B96, B113,
    B122, B127, B131, B154, B157, B159,
    B162, B178, D7, F1
Veterinarians, A97

Veterinary medicine, A97, C6, D15, E9,
    E24, F27, G22, G44, G68, G89
Videotapes, A13
Vision, A65, A174, B158
Vitamin therapy, A136
Vitamins, F7, G11
Vocational nurses *see* Nurses, vocational

Weight reduction, A200
    see also Obesity
Women, A62, A169, B27, B82, E34
World health, A23

X-rays
    technology, A40, A86